The Book of Stars Who Quit Drinking / John Soforic
Wealthy Bookheads Publishing
979-8-9928960-7-7

This is a Nonprofit Book!

The stars who quit drinking were not paid for the personal statements in this book. They spoke for altruistic reasons, sharing their stories to help others who may be struggling to quit drinking. In keeping with their example, **the author will retain no profits from the sale of his book.** All royalties will be recycled into promotions to expose it to others who need these testimonies on the other side of booze. Thank you in advance for your purchase, reviews, and word-of-mouth referrals. Your support is deeply appreciated.

The Book of Stars
Who Quit Drinking

Why They Stop Drinking
Alcohol in Their Own Words

John Soforic

Disclaimer

Why This Book Changes Lives

Why this book? I was inspired by Tony Robbins to create a book of famous people who broke up with booze. In his classic *Awaken the Giant Within*, he wisely advises us to find new references if we want to build new beliefs. Our cultural beliefs about alcohol are deeply entrenched; we have plenty of references about the upside of drinking. It can be fun, exciting, social, sophisticated, sexy, and relaxing. This book shows a different side of the story—providing contrasting references from the most gifted, successful, and famous among us—to support new beliefs and convictions about alcohol. In these pages, you will see common themes that reveal the true nature of the most socially accepted mind-altering drug in history. That said, the stars in this book did not seek inclusion in these pages. I just went looking for them. I spent hours daily for a full year on tedious research. If the quotes aren't perfect, know that I did my best. And while these stars once spoke publicly about their decision to break up with booze, their one-time choice doesn't obligate them to a lifetime commitment. We human beings are all prone to setbacks, changes of mind, and relapse. This book isn't really about the people as much as the poison. It's about alcohol and how this intoxicating chemical can play tricks on even the greatest among us. In this anthology, you will meet extraordinary people who once decided to break up with booze. Let their words shed light on the shadowy side of enjoying a drink for joy or relief. Educate yourself with new references.

Dedication

To all the stars who quit drinking who spoke about this personal decision: your stories will surely help generations to come. You deserve honor, respect, and admiration. You also deserve to be removed from this quote book by contacting me at john@wealthygardener.com. For now, thank you for your vulnerability and courage in speaking publicly about your decision to break up with booze. You didn't have to say a thing. **Thank you for saying it.**

About the Author

I assembled quotes from many stars who quit drinking to put a nail in the coffin of my own drinking tendency. I wrote in past books about the straight edge advantage; I wrote about avoiding vices that feel good in the moment but harm us in the long run. Since the age of 30 (well past my college years, when I was the social coordinator of a wild fraternity), I always believed in abstinence. But still, I would occasionally cheat. Like when I finished my last book, I celebrated with several beers on a boat and felt the euphoria of alcohol for hours in the sun. But then I felt worse, slept poorly, and woke up with a hangover. At other times, when I felt tired, bored, or stressed, I used a glass of wine to take the edge off. I liked the buzz of wine. But one glass was never enough, and then I'd sleep poorly and wake up with remorse. What the heck? I was a nondrinker who cheated mindlessly, albeit infrequently, against my deepest values. No big deal, maybe, but still I felt the inexplicable pull to do something I didn't want to do. So I studied testimonies of famous people to learn more about the mysterious lure of alcohol and the other side of drinking. This task turned into this book, which, in turn, slowly built a firmer foundation in my own belief system to avoid drinking for pleasure and escape. It helped me get clear. I hope it helps you.

It's hard to change your habits if you never change the underlying beliefs that led to your past behavior.

James Clear

We can develop a belief about anything if we just find enough legs—reference experiences—to build it up. Think of your beliefs as a tabletop, and the legs are your references to support it. In other words, start with the basic belief, and reinforce your belief by adding new and more powerful references to uphold it.

Tony Robbins

One day you'll tell your story of how you overcame what you went through, and it will be someone else's survival guide.

Brené Brown

Table of Contents

Preface: What They All Say

Get ready to meet the most beautiful, charming, gifted, rich, famous, and envied people in the world. These stars who quit drinking come from all professions, backgrounds, and social environments. Some of them quit drinking just to feel better in the mornings. Some of them stopped drinking to eliminate a destructive addiction. Some of them never engaged in drinking at all. What these big personalities all tell us—every single one of them quoted herein—is that life is better without booze. This book will show you why. In assembling this book of stars who quit drinking, I've developed an overwhelming empathy for their struggles and an admiration for their triumphs that I did not expect when I began. I found that no matter how glamorous stardom appears, the people we call stars are, indeed, real people. It seems that stardom doesn't relieve stress but rather amplifies it. Fame causes pressures that most of us could never imagine as we sit and watch as spectators. Of course, alcohol takes the edge off; it relieves pain, makes people feel relaxed, funny, sexy, outgoing, euphoric, and sophisticated. So why in the world would any sane person ever want to quit? The answer to this question varies greatly, as you will discover in these pages. But regardless of the reasons to quit drinking, the stars share one common conclusion: they all tell us that life is better without booze.

1. Quotes on the Physical Side

Sleep, Mornings, Hangovers, Energy

I did a sober month — all my girlfriends did it, we all did it together — and I just never went back to it. It felt great, I felt like I looked great. Not that I was a heavy drinker — I wasn't someone who got drunk — but even like two glasses of wine at a girl's night out dinner, I would feel it the next morning. I just didn't really feel the need or desire to go back to it. It wasn't really a choice or a thought, it was just, 'Yeah, I guess I don't drink anymore.' ... I felt better, so I stopped.

Kelly Ripa

I enjoyed it, but the days after drinking were just too rough. If you're an ambitious person and you want to do well in life, you want your body to work well. It's when you're in the gym that you notice feeling better. I haven't had any bad days since I quit drinking. That alone is worth it.

Joe Rogan

I hate shitty sleep more than I enjoy the marginal benefit of being buzzed. I never want to sacrifice tomorrow. I quit drinking even 1 or 2. It affects my gut and any inflammation is noticeable to me. It affects my poise and posture. I feel less powerful in this state. Ultimately it's a distraction.

Alex Hormozi

It became obvious that I had tried everything to feel better. But the one thing I had not done was to stop drinking. So I did and, thank goodness, everything started to get better from there. I burn 75% brighter since I stopped drinking.

Allie Bailey

I woke up and I was like, 'I probably shouldn't drink if I'm going to feel this dreadful.' I started this year doing dry Jan, and just carried on being sober and exercising. I lost like 50 pounds.

Ed Sheeran

When I was drinking, my sleep was awful. My sleep still is a bit hit and miss, but I'm hardly ever up in the night now. Throughout my drinking life, I would wake in the early hours of the morning with my heart racing and my mind in overdrive. One of the considerable advantages of not drinking is the improved quality of life as your broken sleeping patterns repair and you begin to catch up on the lost sleep. This will have a phenomenal impact on your quality of life.

William Porter

I gave up drinking for six months after my divorce because I was just so fed up of feeling so hungover and so anxious. I stopped drinking and I started working out lots and stuff like that to keep me centered. Part of my journey to finding myself again is stopping drinking.

Adele

I understood that other things are way more important than drinking, no matter how fun it gets. Every hangover steals a day. Alcohol is an addictive depressant, and even in moderation that reality doesn't change. You don't have to be a 'problem drinker' for alcohol to affect you adversely. If you drink, it's not fun to work out the next day.

Jocko Willink

My day began with sending my kids off to school and heading to the office — usually with a mild hangover. I can look back on those hangovers now as my body's ultimate cry for help. My body was begging me to listen all this time.

Celeste Yvonne

If you've never quit drinking for 10 days, you don't really know what your face looks like. I didn't realize how much your body and your life changes when it's not in your life every day. You have more mental clarity I think. And you're less bloated. You don't have that puffiness that everyone has when they drink. It's nice to wake up with clarity and to take a break from the bloat.

Chelsea Handler

I stopped drinking about three years ago. Alcohol was not going well with me physically. Just, it was not working anymore. It affects everything, and that's part of the reason why I stopped, because even if you're going out a couple of times a week and you're drinking, it was starting to affect me throughout the week. It wouldn't be necessarily a hangover, but it definitely dimmed my energy. I didn't feel as good. It was affecting anxiety. So, I haven't missed it.

Sanaa Lathan

The mornings are way better. Way better. I mean, literally you do not sleep if you have too much alcohol in your system. Your body's not sleeping. You're just sedated.

Charlie Kirk

I stopped drinking because it actually was making me ill. It was affecting my brain in the worst way. I wasn't an alcoholic or anything like that, but it was clearly affecting what I do. I was annoyed I hadn't been getting enough done, hangovers were taking over.

Calvin Harris

So by going sober, I was more productive, which made me happier, and it happened pretty much straight away. Saturday and Sunday mornings actually existed for me now. I had more attention and better focus. I was able to put my mind onto a single task for a long time, and I like getting things done and being productive—that's a source of happiness for me.

Chris Williamson

It is now pretty definitively clear that no amount of alcohol is good for you. Since I stopped drinking, I feel much better. At least for me, it's easier to either have a habit or not have it, than try to straddle.

Marc Andreessen

When you're having fifteen or twenty drinks a week, you're pretty much constantly in a state of being either drunk or hungover. You don't really realize the degree of damage that you're causing to yourself. But when you cut back and you're only having a few drinks each week, you open up enough gaps of clarity in your day to notice how fucking terrible you feel when you have a drink. Even just one drink—one fucking drink—and it can ruin a whole weekend.

Mark Manson

If you drink at night, and if you want to be productive the next morning, this morning starts last night, and it starts by going to bed at a reasonable time sober. When you're a drunk, what you're doing is you're borrowing tomorrow's dopamine tonight.

Arthur Brooks

I'm enjoying sober life, not missing the 'hanxiety.' I'm feeling more energized, my skin is looking great and I'm sleeping much better. Positives for me really are the time that I've got back, the time that I'm not spent hungover.

Millie Mackintosh

I used to always be hungover until I quit drinking. Now I don't drink, I don't smoke, I don't do drugs. I drink caffeine, I play tennis, I take care of my son. I have no desire to have a drink whatsoever. I was a highly functioning alcoholic. I am much happier not drinking.

Tom Ford

When I stopped drinking it immediately helped alleviate certain problems for me, like crippling hangovers, insomnia, binge eating, constant feelings of shame and regret, as well as some of my more dangerous self-harming behaviors.

Hayley Gibson

When I finally got sober, I took stock of the years I'd spent damaging my body and I decided to take a radically different approach: I'd nurture it instead. I wanted to get healthier and live a better lifestyle. That was a big part of making some healthy choices for myself — choices like what I put in my body, how much sleep I get. And I've been a runner for the past 11 years.

Gregory Gourdet

I quit drinking 25 years ago. Someone dared me to quit drinking for a month, just some silly challenge we were doing. I felt great, and then I was just kind of like, I don't need this in my life. I didn't need alcohol in my life kind of muddying up my weekends. And so I removed that factor entirely, and it certainly has made my life better.

Amber Mac

I'd come to a point in my life where I just felt like I'd had enough. I put a lot of effort into my well-being through diet and exercising, though didn't apply the same discipline to alcohol. I didn't like the way it made me feel anymore. I was determined never to have another hangover in my life because they are such a waste of time. Having a break from alcohol was one of the best things I've ever done. After my year off alcohol, I now drink with awareness and I don't let situations control whether I have a drink or not. My energy levels are much higher, my sleep is better, and I feel like I have more time in the day.

Sarah Jane Clarke

I don't think I really crossed that proverbial line to alcoholic drinking until my late thirties. As I got older and was raising kids, I could definitely start to see that my disease was starting to progress. I started to hide my drinking. I started to drink more than my girlfriends and more often, too.

Carrie Bates

I knew in college that I had an issue with alcohol that just progressed. I was a blackout drinker from the start. I always was hung over. I had blackouts. I had to call in sick.

Kathryn Burgum

I gained lots of weight between ages 18 20 because I was drinking alcohol at night. Alcohol has lots of calories and that does not help. I started taking care of my body much more carefully than I used to. I don't smoke. I don't drink. And I eat healthy. Sobriety was the best gift I ever gave myself. It is more important than Olympic gold.

Oksana Baiul

After gaining weight during the summer, on July 15 I got off the boat and I said, 'That is it. I'm not having any sugar, any carbs, any alcohol.' I thought for maybe two, three weeks… But then I was losing weight and I felt so good, I'm like, 'Why would I go back to that?' I noticed such a difference in my skin and how I felt. The truth is I don't miss it at all. I feel fantastic, so I don't see the point right now. I want to wake up every day feeling my best, mentally and physically strong enough to face whatever comes my way.

Kyle Richards

I used to be a night person but now I go to bed at 11 pm and get up at 8 am. I got tired of feeling like Dracula. I wanted to see some daylight, and not just at six o'clock in the morning. I take care of myself now, I'm a good girl. I go to bed, I drink lots of water, not too much coffee, and I'm trying to cut down on cigarettes. I like to start my day with tea and meditation, followed by some Pilates or yoga. I'm a bit groggy in the afternoon if I don't get eight hours sleep.

Kate Moss

These days I stay sober with routine. I work out every day, try to eat right and drink a lot of water, and I make time to take care of myself.

Mary J. Blige

I'm much happier now, and alcohol is just not a part of my life the way it used to be. It's nice to wake up and actually remember the night before.

Ellie Goulding

Once I saw the scans of my brain, it became a lot harder to pick up the glass. I realized I could have a glass of Champagne tonight if I wanted to. But I don't want to. I feel better without it. My body does not do well with alcohol. I realized that is not a sustainable life for me to live.

Bella Hadid

Even one glass of wine every now and again used to just make me tired. Made my skin tired, made my voice tired. For me, I have to make sure I get sleep and I don't drink, I don't smoke, I will never touch drugs and I have to make sure that I stay sane and happy.

Jessie J

It took me seventeen years to realize alcohol had never done me any favors. For me, going home sober at the end of the night and waking up without a hangover felt like the most wonderfully delicious thing I'd ever experienced.

Holly Whitaker

For years I used alcohol to help me sleep, but the irony is that booze destroys your sleep. You fall into a heavy, boozy sleep, then wake up at 3 a.m. with your heart racing and your mind whirring. I became the sort of woman that my mother would describe as having 'let herself go.' I'm two stone overweight, and most of that is on my belly. It was making me feel depressed, fat, and ill. Then, one day, I said, ENOUGH. I committed to 30 days alcohol free.

Clare Pooley

I was getting to a point where I was living in a way that involved waking up sick and with a lot of shame and just kind of animal confusion. Why couldn't I stop after 6 or 7 drinks? Why didn't I have an 'off' switch when I had that first drink every day? Well, 'Why?' is not a useful question. I got sober when I was 32. I've never had a hangover in these last 37 years, and I've never done anything that I was ashamed of the next day, which is a pretty incredible trade-off.

Anne Lamott

I've never been a big drinker. I don't drink. Do as you wish, but know what you're doing. When you ingest alcohol, you are ingesting a poison, and that poison is converted into an even worse poison in your body. Alcohol is a toxin. Past two drinks a week is when you start seeing some negative health effects in males and females. I invite others to provide studies… if they exist… that alcohol can be beneficial. No consumption… zero consumption… is going to be better for your health than low to moderate consumption of alcohol. The sleep you get after even one drink is vastly diminished.

Andrew Huberman

I'm not in any way, physically or psychologically addicted to alcohol anymore. And yet once you've done something to an addicted level, those neural pathways live on in the brain. Neural pathways in the brain, including addictive pathways, are formed in a similar way to hiking trails. The more a hiking route is used, the smoother, wider and clearer it becomes. It becomes the default, easiest route. Should you need to forge a brand new path through the forest (or form a newborn sober neural pathway), it will be arduous initially. At first, this new path will be narrow, difficult, and slow. Over time, it will become a well-worn, comfortable path. It will be just as easy as the original path.

Catherine Gray

The daily morning habit of the workout breaks the nighttime going out and drinking habit. There is a place for alcohol in life, but you should understand the tradeoffs: hangovers, reduced capacity the next day. If I drink the night before, the morning workout becomes a lot more difficult. The morning workout checkpoint really helped me understand the consequences of consuming alcohol before. Morning workouts helped me stop drinking alcohol.

Naval Ravikant

I hadn't drunk in a while, was healthy, doing my thing, and then I went to Italy on my babymoon and started drinking. I drank way too much and got violently hungover. I threw up 15 times. I was almost crippled for the entire day. It was horrible and because of that I'm never drinking again, and I mean that.

Logan Paul

It's not a big deal for me and I don't gravitate towards it. Nutrition is so important; it's part of the game. It has helped with my recovery, allowed me to sleep better, and helped my body adapt quickly. I myself don't want to drink and I don't want to try.

Mohamed Salah

I struggled with alcohol for years, ruined my body and completely checked out mentally and was going to drink until I couldn't anymore. I was just tired of feeling like crap. Waking up hungover, not remembering what I said or what I did the night before. I just really liked to drink, and drink, and drink, many times until I blacked out. It's poison now. I don't even think about it or need it. I always tell people, if you think you might have a problem, you probably have a problem.

CC Sabathia

I feel much better now that I don't drink and have straightened my life out. I feel like a different person now that I'm sober.

Brett Favre

You want to become a pro footballer, and you're going out drinking and staying out late? It doesn't make sense. If you look after yourself and you don't drink... then you feel ready for the game at the weekend. Everyone knows I don't drink alcohol. That's probably why I'm still playing to be honest.

Jermain Defoe

I was drinking every day, showing up to practices hungover, and I was close to losing everything – my career, my health, my relationships. It was March 11, the day I got sober. It was the best decision I ever made. It saved my life. Without my sobriety, I wouldn't be here right now.

Maxx Crosby

No more hangovers, no more chaos, just getting on with life. I haven't had a drink for 19 years. I just don't even think about drinking anymore.

Robbie Williams

I just really got to a point where I wasn't enjoying it anymore. The hangovers were just brutal... it was like my body was being torn apart from the inside out. You'd wake up feeling like you'd been hit by a truck.

Slash

I had a hangover for pretty much 15 years. I didn't want to live in that haze anymore. I am not a preacher. I don't want to stand on a soapbox and tell people, 'Don't drink. Don't use drugs.' But I'm sober and I'm happy being sober. I like that I'm very lucid and clear.

Nikki Sixx

I got tired of being sick, I got tired of feeling like I didn't have a reason to wake up in the morning. What I've realized along the way is that it's one day at a time. It's how am I showing up today?

Macklemore

I'd plan my life around a hangover: 'The Misfits are playing in town Friday night, so Saturday is hangover day.' I lost a lot of days in my life.

James Hetfield

Several doctors had questioned me about why my liver was larger than it needed to be, so I knew I was in trouble one way or the other. I started drinking when I was like 12 and didn't stop until I was in my thirties. I was drinking heavily in those days — that may have provided some fuel for misery.

David Letterman

I was at a point in my life where it was like, this has got to stop, because my hangovers were getting so ridiculous and debilitating for a whole day. I was gonna get a DUI which was going to financially destroy me and potentially physically destroy me or others.

Nikki Glaser

I would always rather wake up early and go for a run. I'd rather work. I hate losing a day to something so dumb.

Casey Neistat

Removing alcohol from my life helped me quit cigarettes. It helped me reverse health conditions. My new addiction is running. I run three miles every day.

Travis Barker

I have no use for alcohol. I never had a drink in my life.

Jackie Robinson

I don't have that story to tell of just imploding. I got up in the morning. It just was taking a toll. I could feel it extracting a pound of flesh. I felt I was poisoning myself by degrees. When you have a six-month-clean liver, it's kind of like a superpower.

Ben Harper

For every hour of fun, I had a week of misery that I put on myself. Most of the time, I just felt like shit. I felt like I had a serious illness when I wasn't drunk. Now if I woke up one morning feeling like I did ten years ago, every day, I would think I was dying and I would immediately go to the emergency room. But when it was a hangover, I thought I deserved it, so I just put up with it. I was drinking a lot—that was my main problem.

Jason Isbell

I got sober at 19. I never had a hangover again, which was awesome. I feel like self-care is now finally a cool thing. When before, it was like you're a freak. I don't drink at all.

Soko

I'm 72 years of age. I don't drink alcohol anymore. I don't smoke tobacco. I don't use drugs. I'm doing good right now. And I think that says a lot for why I'm still here. Most of the people that I drank with are dead. And the ones that aren't, that still continue to drink, are going to be dead soon. It's not a happy ending.

Ozzy Osbourne

You get addicted to being sober, that's all. I went through the whole alcohol and drug thing 35 years ago. I stopped doing everything, and I've never been in better shape. If I hadn't stopped, I would have been gone. It was one of those things where my body and everything else says: 'This is it, make a choice. When I was drinking, I had to have another one and another one and another one.

Alice Cooper

I've never seen any life transformation that didn't begin with the person in question finally getting tired of their own bullshit. I wrote books when I had hangovers. It's just that I don't want to anymore.

Elizabeth Gilbert

Don't know if sobriety is forever or not but I can't imagine going back to how things were. I like waking up with no hangover or embarrassment. I like waking up with no night terrors and panic attacks from liquor.

Ari Lennox

One of my best decisions that I ever made in my life was to stop drinking. I feel amazing physically and mentally. I look 10 times better than I did four years ago.

Allen Iverson

I like to go to bed at 10pm, or 10.30pm, because I like to wake up at 7am. I'm a goodie two shoes, like a control freak or something. I'm like one glass of wine and I'm good. I've never been hung over.

Mandy Moore

In 1983, I began the journey to sobriety, utilizing 12 step programs as well as vigorous exercise. Eventually, that sort of just scours the devil out of you, so that's the best practical advice I can give — sweat it out. It's the one piece of advice I give to people in recovery: You've got to start moving. It's the only way to get your nervous system back. For years I had to have three hours of exercise every day, no matter what. It was the only way I could stand to be in my own skin.

James Taylor

I was sick of waking up with a dry throat, sick of feeling bloated and sick of the decisions I make on it. Sobriety for me is more than never having a hangover. It's being fully present for every moment, it's being the healthiest version of myself, and it's knowing I will never hurt anyone important to me ever again. I want to feel clear.

Jack Harlow

The paparazzi photos following the 2022 Burning Man festival gave me a wake-up call and how it, in part, encouraged me to get sober. I hadn't slept. I was not okay. It's heartbreaking because I thought I was having fun, but at some point it was like, 'Okay, I don't look well.' Sometimes you need a reality check, so in a way those pictures were something to be grateful for.

Cara Delevingne

There's nothing I could drink to improve the way I'm feeling right now. I certainly don't miss anxiously waking up in the middle of the night after drinking. Although it required discipline and persistence, the bottom line is you can't be well and present in your life if you're not present and well, and alcohol doesn't really support that.

Elle MacPherson

I don't want to wake up feeling groggy. I want to wake up feeling ready. I just don't want to drink. I want to be in control of myself and my decisions.

Zendaya

The way I drink leads to brutal, days long hangovers. My last hangover lasted for five days. I'd earned it: it was a day drinking session with friends that went into an evening birthday party with one of my drinking buddies. I will never be that person who can nurse a glass of wine throughout an entire evening. Deep down I knew alcohol wasn't for me, and once I accepted that, 'none at all' made sense.

Anne Hathaway

Eliminating alcohol has significantly impacted my fitness journey, and I'm feeling healthier now than I did in my 30s. It's amazing how these changes start to compound—not just physically, but also in how I show up every day. I had no idea that cutting even the occasional drink could have such a significant impact.

Steven Bartlett

I would start to get these hangovers that were debilitating. I was 33, and my wife was pregnant with our fourth child, and I was fairly functional. I mean, I did a daily TV show, was fairly well known, kind of famous actually at that point—so, you know, I was kind of killing it. I don't understand it all, really—but your body responds to alcohol differently as you age.

Tucker Carlson

I'd probably be dead by now if I hadn't stopped drinking. The drinking was what would kick my butt for a long time. ... I became concerned about my health after seeing how drinking hurt other former players. Quitting gave me a chance to survive and get healthier.

Joe Namath

I don't drink coffee or alcohol... they're bad for my body.

Bruce Lee

I think I have pancreatic cancer because for most of my life, though I was never a drunk, I drank too much. And if you do that, even if you think you're too strong to get anything, somehow you're going to pay.

Michael Landon

Here's a nice little side effect of Dry January. These jeans that I'm wearing were so tight a few months ago that I couldn't comfortably button them. Now, they're so loose it's time for me to go down a size.

Valerie Bertinelli

And I think, when I was with the Ryan White family in Indianapolis when Ryan died, and I played the funeral, and I was probably at the height of my unhappiness. If you look back at footage of me there, I looked like a 75-year-old white-haired man, about 300-pound man playing the piano. And I was really ashamed of myself.

Elton John

I just got a point where I'd had enough. I didn't enjoy being completely inebriated, and it probably created more problems in my life than I needed. I don't need it now. I used to get offstage and be so wound up and adrenalized that I needed something to calm down to go to sleep. But I realized when you're drinking yourself to sleep, you're not really sleeping. You're just passing out.

Billy Joel

I realized that I didn't want to wake up feeling like that anymore. One or two drinks was never enough for me. I was a foot-on-the-floor-all-the-way drinker, so it had to go. I don't miss it. Now it's as if I never had a drink in my life.

Gerard Butler

Are there days I'm sitting on the golf course or sitting on my patio and would like to have a beer? Yeah. But I have a year left in my career. If I really want it bad enough, I will make that sacrifice.. My body fat has dropped significantly, and I'm leaner than I've ever been. The performances are there because I worked, recovered, slept and took care of myself more than I ever had. I can really tell the difference with my body, sort of not carrying that weight on my back.

Michael Phelps

I don't drink alcohol and I don't need an energy drink. I have never missed a session at the gym, a meeting, or an early morning flight because I had too much to drink the night before.

50 Cent

When I'm not drinking, I'm sleeping much better. You have got to take care of this only vehicle you got, right?" If others want to drink, that's their choice; I'm happy with my herbal tea.

Gisele Bündchen

I don't know if I'm going to drink again. Since I've stopped drinking, I've just been feeling so much better, so much more clarity. I sleep better. I wake up in the morning and I can still get up at 5 a.m. I've always been looking for how do you get that extra 1%.

Lewis Hamilton

These are pictures from huge moments in life where my eyes just look... gone. Some are from real work shoots, some just beach days with the family. While I honestly STILL don't know if I'll never have a drink again, I do know I never want to be that way again. I was done with making a fool of myself in public, tired of hangovers, and unable to sleep, so I stopped drinking. I know I like myself better sober, I get more done, and I feel physically better without alcohol. I was, point blank, just drinking too much.

Chrissy Teigen

2. Quotes on the Emotional Side

Happiness, Anxiety, Feelings, Discomfort

For two to three days after I would drink, I'd be more emotional. I'd get crankier, more excited, more embarrassed. But since quitting drinking entirely, I find that I am on an incredibly even keel. This has been an unexpected boon for my productivity and work. There's much less energy being spent on trying to manage my emotions and much more energy being invested into creativity.

Mark Manson

I was boozing too much. It's just become a problem. I didn't want to live that way anymore. I was running from feelings. I was running to things to avoid, to avoid tough feelings, painful feelings. I just didn't know how to deal with them and looking for anything to use for escape. I guess it was difficult feelings. I don't know how better to describe it. You either deny your feelings all of your life or you answer them. That's the thing about becoming un-numb. I've got my feelings in my fingertips again.

Brad Pitt

I treated alcohol like it was my friend. It made me feel less nervous, less shy, less scared. But it wasn't my friend, it was poison. It was killing me and everybody around me could see it except me. I was a classic self-medicator, that's what alcoholics do. I was using booze to try to fill up a hole in my life. It never works, it just makes the hole bigger. You wake up feeling worse and then you drink again.

Billy Joel

I always drank, from when it was legal for me to drink. And there was never a time for me when the goal wasn't to get as hammered as I could possibly afford to. But when the alcohol wears off, so does the happiness, and the anxiety and depression return.

Stephen King

I feel whole again. There's a way of dealing with hardships that are healthier than going out. Addiction isn't about the drinking. It's about what you're trying to escape. I feel better not drinking. It's more fun.

Lindsay Lohan

I'm a big believer in taking breaks from alcohol for many reasons. I started with a month, and then I just didn't want to go back. You realize how much the 'hangxiety' was affecting your mental health. I worked out it was social anxiety that really made me use alcohol to take the edge off of my feelings. I didn't like the way alcohol made me feel anymore. I just wanted to be present.

Sarah Jane Clarke

Fame doesn't protect you from pain; if anything, it amplifies it. I never drank while I was working or preparing. I would clean up, go back to work — I could do both. However many months of shooting, bang, it's time to go. Then, boom. Three months of wine. Two bottle a day.

Denzel Washington

Drinking would give me anxiety the next day. I was not someone who could just go out and drink and have fun and be happy. Alcohol made me feel depressed the next day no matter how fun the night before was. And honestly, life is going to throw us some difficult days. I certainly don't need to be adding any extra ones to that list. The next day I was always feeling down. I want to wake up every day feeling my best, mentally and physically strong enough to face whatever comes my way. I'm exercising and not drinking, because guess what, even if I have two glasses of wine, the next day I feel down and depressed. I can't afford to be depressed right now.

Kyle Richards

When people ask me when I knew it was time to quit drinking, I often say: when the shame of my drinking became louder than the relief it gave me. I was very much entranced by the mommy wine culture, and

I used that culture to self-medicate. I needed an outlet and I needed a way to escape. The 'mommy needs wine' narrative gaslights women by implying the mental load they carry is something a few drinks can fix. I think one of the greatest disservices of our times is the notion that a mother's stress is something she should drink away. I've been sober for eight years now, and truly, the first year was 365 days of inner turmoil as I tried to learn a new way of life, to cope, and to function. I used to drink to numb my brain, my heart, my feelings. Now I feel everything, and recognize what my body is trying to tell me. I will never drink again. I don't ever want to drink again.

Celeste Yvonne

After sobriety, I learned that only people who truly know themselves can be with themselves in solitude. I used alcohol to manage my anxiety, my depression, my loneliness, my boredom, my hunger, my exhaustion, my rage, my joy—every feeling I didn't know how to sit with. My drinking wasn't cute or quirky; it was obliteration. I drank to disappear.

Holly Whitaker

I wasn't raised with the skills and emotional practice needed to 'lean into discomfort,' so over time I basically became a take-the-edge-off-aholic. We can anesthetize with a whole bunch of stuff including alcohol. We can take the edge off emotional pain with alcohol, drugs, food, sex, relationships, money, work, caretaking, gambling, staying busy, affairs, chaos, shopping, planning, perfectionism, constant change, and the Internet. But pain is unrelenting. It will get our attention. Despite our attempts to drown it in addiction, pain will find a way to make itself known.

Brené Brown

I used to drink because I was nervous to be around people. I don't need that anymore. I stopped drinking because I wanted to choose my life, not have alcohol choose it for me. I couldn't function sober. And for a long time, I didn't want to say that out loud.

Nikki Glaser

Anxiety and alcohol really do not mix. You're adding alcohol in to try and numb those feelings of anxiety – and it's like pouring lighter fluid on a flame. I'd say the gift is also the emotional sobriety that you get when you stop drinking the toxic substance. Sobriety has been the ultimate act of self-love. It has been messy and hard and uncomfortable at times but it has transformed me in ways I never thought possible. It has given me back a life I actually want to live and more importantly it has given me back myself.

Millie Mackintosh

I suppose I began to drink heavily after I'd realized that the things I'd wanted most in life for myself and my writing, and my wife and children, were simply not going to happen. It's very painful to think about some of the things that happened back then.

Raymond Carver

In all my life, I never drank for the sake of drinking. It was always a response to some kind of emotional difficulty I was going through. If I'm drinking for emotional reasons, that's when there's a problem.

Patrick Swayze

The best thing about recovery is that you get your feelings back. The worst thing about recovery is, you get your feelings back. We think that alcohol helps when we're going through a traumatic time, but actually being sober makes you so much stronger and more able to cope. The only thing I knew that could take the edge off that immense fear was alcohol. But I got myself sorted out. I've spent decades not growing, learning or moving forward, but desperately treading water in a sea of Sauvignon Blanc. It takes a long time to recondition your mind to not go to that solution.

Clare Pooley

I hate feelings. Why does sobriety have to come with feelings? One minute I feel excited, the next I feel terrified. One minute I feel like everything is possible, the next I feel like nothing is possible.

Augusten Burroughs

In some deep and important personal respects you stop growing when you start drinking alcoholically. The drink stunts you. I drank when I was happy and I drank when I was anxious and I drank when I was bored and I drank when I was depressed, which was often. My favorite line was, I'll drink less when things get better. The real struggle is about you: you, a person who has to learn to live in the real world, to inhabit her own skin, to know her own heart, to stop waiting for life to begin. Drinking is a form of self-medication. Sobriety is less about 'getting better' in a clear, linear sense than it is about subjecting yourself to change, to the inevitable ups and downs that accompany growth.

Caroline Knapp

After sobriety, I learned that only people who truly know themselves can be with themselves in solitude. I used alcohol to manage my anxiety, my depression, my loneliness, my boredom, my hunger, my exhaustion, my rage, my joy—every feeling I didn't know how to sit with. My drinking wasn't cute or quirky; it was obliteration. I drank to disappear.

Holly Whitaker

I want to make sure that every single thing I feel is real. I want no masking. I want nothing to mask my ability to feel fear, to overcome fear, whatever it may be. And I say that people who drink are trying to hide. I think of it as a masking agent, so that your mind doesn't have to work a hard. That means I'm losing.

David Goggins

Becoming sober is like recovering from frostbite. The process of defrosting is excruciatingly painful. You have been so numb for so long. Sadness, loss, fear, anger, all of these things that you have been numbing with the booze, you start to FEEL them for the first time. And it's horrific at first, to tell you the damn truth. It's just a real big reckoning with all the things you've been trying to keep beneath the surface. The thing that I tried to do for so long is numb out the brutal. That's what addiction is — it's a hiding place from pain and numbing out. If you numb the brutal, you don't get to experience the beautiful.

Glennon Doyle

I started drinking every day. I'd come home from work and start to drink. Quitting is hard because you've taught yourself, 'This is the only way to ease my pain.' I'm in pain; this thing will make it better.'

Ben Affleck

Alcohol was a way I could shut my thoughts up and lose myself for hours, for days, and I didn't have to face how much I really disliked myself. And when you're sober it is unfiltered reality all day every day. You don't get a brain break. It is an act of rebellion to remain present, to go against society's desire for you to numb yourself, to look away. But we must not look away. But now, I can move through the world with so much more freedom and independence. I'm so much more in tune with what I want, what I like and what I want to make.

Florence Welch

I did a full thirty days, I fully surrendered. I learned more about myself than I ever thought was possible. And I've been sober ever since. Alcohol makes you feel like you're having fun, but it's a lie. It's just numbing you out. It takes everything away, and gives you nothing. When you get sober, it's like you've been given your life back. You can actually see and feel things again. It's a whole new world.

Slash

I stopped drinking. That's one great way of really sort of getting to know yourself is being sober, just drinking water and being sober as anything. Once I realized I had a lot of work to do on myself, I stopped drinking and started working out lots to keep me sort of centered.

Adele

I used to think it was the world, but now I think it's me. I never went out when I was in high school or college. I was pathologically shy, and because of that I was drunk all the time. My entire life I found ways to self-medicate. I was anxious and hypochondriacal and an alcoholic, and many, many other things that made me different from other people.

David Letterman

I knew how to drink just enough to remove myself from reality, to disconnect from feelings. I was very sad. I was very scared. Since a very young age, I always felt alone and misunderstood. So as a teenager, I found alcohol which of course shut my brain off. And it worked for me for a while, until it turned really dark. It was me trying to fix something that was broken inside of me. It's been a crazy journey, but I'm very grateful. I just feel safe in my body again. I wouldn't give this feeling up for anything.

Lucy Hale

Booze was preventing me from being fully present in my life. What I actually needed was to learn how to feel everything I'd been using alcohol to numb. If I'm drinking to suppress negative emotions, when the alcohol wears off and the hangover sets in, it all comes back feeling 10 times more overwhelming. Every time I took a longer break from drinking I realized how much better I felt without alcohol.

Ruby Warrington

If sugar didn't make me feel better, I wouldn't use it. If caffeine didn't make me feel better, I wouldn't use it. If alcohol and drugs didn't make me feel different and better, I wouldn't use them. The reason we are living in <u>such</u> a time of mass addiction is because all of those things work to make you feel better. I don't need alcohol and drugs to alter my consciousness … It's been about six-and-a-half years of not using anyone or anything to alter my mood or mind — and that's a miracle.

Elizabeth Gilbert

I'm just going to say something for the first time in a long time: I have not had a drink of alcohol in two and a half years. Why do we drink, you know? To be free of pain, to be free of shyness — it's like that liquid courage. It was something that I realized just did not serve me in my life.

Pink

It's taken years — and it will probably be a lifetime — of unraveling how far I had strayed from my inner compass. I suspect there was a lot of self-medication going on. Drinking and drugging had turned into a full-time job. I wasn't showing up for the rest of my life. It wasn't a good picture. I couldn't see at the time how much I had lost.

Trey Anastasio

The sobriety journey is really about reparenting yourself. It's about learning how to process feelings, because drugs and alcohol are a symptom of a much deeper issue. People talked about numbing the discomfort of being in their own skin, and then having to face themselves in the cold light of sobriety – that was my story too. My point is you have to be present enough to understand when it's time to give certain things up, but you also need tools to know how to deal with being present. Sometimes you get really bored, sometimes you have a lot of pain, a lot of loneliness, but you need the tools to deal with that otherwise you're gonna be in a lot of pain.

RuPaul

I used alcohol to create a fake, more confident version of myself, but that feeling was an illusion. Drinking became my tool for panic and anxiety, until the hangovers and fear lasted into the next night. Getting sober let me wake up clear, present, and able to feel my life instead of numbing it.

Rumer Willis

I was drinking to escape discomfort—emotional, spiritual, existential. Alcohol was my anesthetic. I was a kid who was very awkward and who had difficulty making friends and who was a loner and an isolator. I was generally insecure, and feeling like everybody had things figured out except me. And I think from the very first time I drank, there was a very palpable, visceral sense of this being a solution. Suddenly feeling comfortable in my own skin for the first time —and so I drank to excess the very first time that I drank. It was always to excess, and I was always the guy who was the last guy to leave the party and the most drunk and all of that. I finally found something that allowed me to talk to a girl at a party and crack a joke, and feel somewhat self-assured, albeit medically enhanced. And that worked for quite some time, until it stopped working.

Rich Roll

I think it's more important to focus on the quality of the life that you're living and how you're living life to the fullest. Drinking took away the anxiety I felt about trying to be a perfect partner, mother, model and businesswoman. But it's very difficult to get to know yourself if you're numbing yourself. Sobriety is a decision that I've never regretted.

Elle MacPherson

If you're drinking not to feel something, that's a red flag. I was drinking to escape an enormous unhappiness and huge anxiety, and the problem is that when you numb the bad things, you also numb the good.

Elizabeth Vargas

One thing that addiction does is, it freezes you. You don't develop, you don't learn the skills by trial and error of having experiences and learning from them, and finding out what it is you want, and how to go about getting it, by relating with other people. I found out I hadn't learned any skills or social cues or the habits you're supposed to pick up between 18 and 35. When you're addicted, you short-circuit all those life lessons.

James Taylor

I was self-medicating with alcohol. That's what I thought would make me happy and get out of that depression. When I would wake up the next day after a night like that, you are left staring at the ceiling by yourself, and in that depression and back in that hole. As much as I loved football, there was something else in college and high school that I got really good at, and that was partying. As things started to go bad in my football life, I turned to something else that I was really good at. Where did that get me except out of the NFL?

Johnny Manziel

Alcohol abuse began when I felt empty despite having everything I thought I wanted. Here you are with this massive void and massive lack of self-love and you're doing all these things — sports, making a bunch of money, hooking up with girls, drinking, doing drugs — to try to fill that void... and really it's never going to work. The alcohol and all that actually just makes it deeper. Walking away from it was the hardest, but the best, decision I made.

Jake Paul

Looking around, everyone seemed so happy. But for me, I was depressed. I felt beaten down and out of ideas for how to manage my life. I always thought one more drink, then I would be happy. Alcohol felt like a shortcut to relief. Not happiness. Not healing. Relief. Sometimes it feels harder because now I don't have anything to distract me or to numb the pain when life throws me an uppercut.

Kevin Kreider

I was just so deeply depressed. That fueled the drinking. When you're depressed you drink more and when you drink more you get more depressed. I realized I wasn't drinking to relax. I was drinking to escape. It took me a while maybe to be able to get back to being able to be joyful and silly without alcohol. I am much happier not drinking.

Tom Ford

Early on, however, it also became clear that stopping drinking hadn't solved all of my problems. As much as my alcohol abuse was a gargantuan problem in itself, it was fundamentally a symptom of larger issues.

Hayley Gibson

Often when I was drinking, it was this idea that I'm in charge. I grew up with anxiety and I used alcohol to relieve my fears and insecurities. It got so bad that eventually I ended up in a hospital for mental health.

Jamie Campbell Bower

Inside, I was dying. I remember drinking for the sole reason of not feeling. When I went into treatment in 2012, they asked me, 'What makes you happy?' And I couldn't answer. I had a lot of suicidal ideation while I was under the influence.

Carrie Bates

I grew up, my life had a lot of trauma. I was just drinking because it was basically covering up the pain of poor me. I felt a lot of pain inside and pressure, so I turned to alcohol. The beginning of sobriety was brutal. There was nothing pretty about it. No confidence. No peace. Just survival, one minute at a time. Instead of going to drink, I started finding other things, like just being comfortable in your own skin and being okay.

Oksana Baiul

I genuinely could not cope when my mum died. I got to the point I couldn't turn my brain off, and the wine suffocated everything. I would start with a glass of wine, and before I knew it, that glass would turn into a bottle. I just stopped drinking for the good and the better for me. I prefer me now I'm sober. To feel so free and able day in day out, is a true joy!

Lisa Riley

I couldn't manage my feelings, so I had to take something to manage my feelings. I turned to alcohol as a social lubricant. That helped me at the time until it stopped helping me. My heart is full of gratitude for a life I never could have imagined when I put down alcohol at 25.

Amber Valletta

I dealt with my rapid rise to fame and relentless touring through excessive drinking. I couldn't deal with anything. I was drinking, and I was not really myself. It's only when you come out of that phase you realize you were in trouble. I think I was just trying to figure out who I was. I'm much happier now, and alcohol is just not a part of my life the way it used to be.

Ellie Goulding

I don't feel the need to drink because I know how it will affect me at 3 in the morning when I wake up with horrible anxiety thinking about that one thing I said five years ago when I graduated high school.

Bella Hadid

I numbed myself with alcohol. I thought that running marathons would save me from myself, but it was me that had to do that. Since I have stopped drinking this has flipped itself. I will now do anything, ANYTHING to avoid feeding that emotional pain that has been attempting to kill me for so many years. And that means never drinking again. And that is 100% non-negotiable. I can honestly say, hand on heart, that I will never, ever drink again. There is no doubt in my mind.

Allie Bailey

As soon as I felt that first alcoholic buzz, I was hooked. Who wants to work hard to feel good about yourself when there's a path that's a lot easier? When I drank, I felt like the edges rounded. I felt prettier and smarter, and I didn't have to jump in a cold pool at 5 a.m. to feel that way. Now, almost 40 years after taking my first drink, I've learned that we could all benefit from being patient with ourselves and kind to ourselves. It's never too late for a do-over.

Karlyn Pipes

I'm not really the party person. I don't 'become myself' once I'm drunk. I don't use alcohol to be happy.

Jessie J

Very simply put, if you have a problem, drinking will not solve it. In fact, it can only make it worse. Anything extra at all I just couldn't cope with when I was drinking. Alcohol is an anesthetic and a depressant. Things that are genuinely awful but manageable can transform into the genuinely awful and unbearable if you factor in the depressing after-effects of alcohol consumption.

William Porter

I drink to numb. I drink to forget. I drink to not feel. I drink not to be me. Whenever I had too much to drink, this was my mantra: 'I'm fine.' It was easy to say without slurring, and it was defiant. I didn't know who I would be without alcohol. I didn't know if I would still be fun and funny.

Ann Dowsett Johnston

I needed alcohol to drink away the things that plagued me. Not just my doubts about sex. My self-consciousness, my loneliness, my insecurities, my fears. I drank away all the parts that made me human.

I couldn't understand why the happiness never came, couldn't see the flaw in my thinking, couldn't see that alcohol kept me trapped in a world of illusion, procrastination, paralysis. I lived always in the future, never in the present. Next time, next time! Next time I drank it would be different, next time it would make me feel good again. And all my efforts were doomed, because already drinking hadn't made me feel good in years. I finally understood alcohol was not a cure for pain; it was merely a postponement.

Sarah Hepola

I was medicating myself so I could escape my pain and insecurities. What I did was drink myself to sleep at night. If I wasn't with someone, I was an unhappy girl.

Melanie Griffith

I was resorting to alcohol and drugs to numb the pain. People from the outside looking in would think I was great, but I was in hell. I was in a dark, dark place. Alcohol and drugs had taken over. The more I drank, the more depressed I became. Sobriety didn't come easy. I had to stop running, stop drinking, and finally face myself.

Mary J. Blige

I think I was asleep for a lot of years. I was just self-medicating myself through my problems, through my divorce, through moving out of my house. I was doing all of these speeches, I was supposed to be inspiring people – inspiring people! – and late at night, in my hotel room, I was drinking myself to sleep. In the end, when things spun out of control. I started to use more to counterbalance the pain I was feeling of not knowing how to deal with those emotions. I was out of control.

Abby Wambach

I'm willing to go through pain to preserve my recovery and my spiritual progress. If I have to be in pain, I'll be in pain. I'll be okay. I feel like I was addicted to validation from people long before I was ever addicted to, like, drugs and alcohol.

Darren Waller

Dealing with the effects of childhood abuse and how it affected me in so many ways. Drinking became a part where I just escaped from it and stuffed my feelings down. I used to go and sit in my $2 million dollar home and feel empty. It's all fun, and then it becomes toxic. You're never free; there's always an emptiness inside. You have to allow yourself to be healed on the inside from that brokenness. Then you'll be able to find freedom and have the liberty to enjoy life to the fullest. I have managed to maintain sobriety for over 27 years after battling addiction. True recovery requires a deep, internal change.

Darryl Strawberry

I knew that I was alcohol dependent from the first time I had a drink when I was 14 years old. I drank because it made me feel nothing at all. And that was a lot easier than really dealing with my issues. There was always a reason to drink. Even my very first drink I took was to get away from all the trauma that I was experiencing.

CC Sabathia

I wasn't happy. As much as I had, I had low self-esteem. I didn't feel good about myself. I didn't drink to socialize. I drank to get drunk. I drank to escape. I wanted time to stop. I wanted the world to go away. I wanted instant gratification. I knew I needed help, but after the next drink I didn't need it.

Sugar Ray Leonard

Alcohol had been my release from stress and pressure. The drinking started increasing as years started going on. And then it led to the drugs. I would medicate myself with the drugs and alcohol. Any time I would feel bad or feel good, that was like my scapegoat.

Doc Gooden

When I was drunk or high then I wouldn't think about being depressed. When I was drunk, I'd feel great, like a boxing champion, but when the drink wore off it just left me with a bad hangover and feeling even more depressed. At one point I believed I was being tortured by demons.

Tyson Fury

So you know, any kind of pain, we want to get away from it, and alcohol introduced me to that. I wasn't ready to get sober, because being sober meant not sleeping to me. I was raped in a dark room on a bed, which meant sleeping was not an option because all I could feel was shame and fear and guilt. The direct result of my being abused was that I became a fucking raging, alcoholic lunatic. I turned to drugs, alcohol and gambling as a way to cope and numb the pain.

Theo Fleury

I was dying, I was lost… just mentally I couldn't… I was not happy deep down. It was fun in the moment, but it got worse and worse.

Maxx Crosby

I drank too much, too often, for too long. I had suppressed every emotion in booze. I didn't know who I was. I had to learn absolutely everything, I was a child again so when I sobered up I got to know myself.

Tony Adams

I drank and I took drugs to numb the pain. That was a quick one-way trip into hell and eventually I had to stop drinking. What happens is, when you stop drinking, you're left with the person that you are. And the person who I really was, was depressed and isolated. I didn't know how to socialize. I didn't know how to be a human.

Robbie Williams

If you don't deal with your demons, they will deal with you, and it's gonna hurt. For me, taking away the substance just gave me an honest view of who I had become and then the healing started. Sobriety isn't just about eliminating substances; it's about the ability to be honest with yourself and those around you. When I got sober, a few years later, that was when some of the greatest lessons came.

Nikki Sixx

I finally realized that I was just self-soothing, I was auto regulating using alcohol. I was starting to get a little bit famous and it was destabilizing. None of my friends thought I was an alcoholic, and neither did I. I was really unhappy being an artist and I was getting sicker and sicker.

Sia

I drank for about 25 years getting over the loss of my father, and I took the anger out on myself. You could call it a coping mechanism, but that would be an excuse. I just drank too much. I did a good job at beating myself up sometimes. I can't be my authentic self without sobriety. That and my spiritual life are the only things that can't be taken from me. I wouldn't wish it on my worst enemy, to be in the grip of it. It's hell.

Gary Oldman

I used to think that the alcohol was the way I could access my feelings... but it was completely the opposite. Drinking was a way for me to not deal with things, to hide from the world.

James Hetfield

One of the reasons I drank was because I had issues with anxiety and getting sober enabled me to get a lot of help and support for that — the idea of managing Elton before I got sober would have been utterly terrifying.

David Furnish

I sought things that would put a blanket over my feelings. Numb them down, turn it all off. Things that would bring me down and things that would make me feel less. I was not having fun. I was very scared and uncomfortable and sad. But I didn't know how to name any of those emotions. I was just doing it because that's what you do. Or that's what people around me were doing. It was more like a numbing agent, or an escape mechanism, I suppose. The other fear is that when substances aren't there and I'm alone, I'm going to have confront something even scarier, which is myself and my own consciousness. It's an extremely necessary skill—the ability to be alone and to confront yourself. You can't hide behind substances all the time.

Julien Baker

If you have the slightest amount of self-loathing, when you stop using alcohol, it rears its head a bit higher. The emotional edge that it does take off is real. So living with that, with life in its most raw form, is a bit daunting. Just taking life full on, without that influence, was hard. You're removing the capacity to be present, not just in the bad moments. You're numbing the good feelings. You're numbing everything. It's profoundly selfish.

Ben Harper

I immediately went right to drugs and alcohol in my teens. I don't remember feeling like there was any other way to be happy. I just felt like I was chasing chaos and making my life difficult, all the time thinking I was having fun. But I didn't think it was very good for my life.

Christina Ricci

I was spiraling down a path of real self-destruction and no matter what success I had I just never felt good enough. I had absolutely no value for myself and this self-destructive path really quickly brought me to a real crisis point. Unfortunately, even as we try to submerge our pain deep down inside, it finds a way to bubble up: through addiction. Part of being sober is I don't want to miss a moment of life, of that texture, even if that means being in some pain.

Demi Moore

I had no esteem, because I wasn't doing any esteem(able) acts. I don't have a drinking problem, I have a sobriety problem. I have been abusive to myself and everyone around me for years. I have no excuses for my alcoholism or aggression, only rationalizations.

Shia LaBeouf

Eliminating caffeine and alcohol from your diet is another self-care tip that's essential to lowering anxious feelings. When you're living in a beautiful state, you don't need drugs or alcohol to enjoy your life.

Tony Robbins

What's tough is having to change… having to not have a beer if you need it … Owning angst. Sometimes the hardest part isn't quitting, it's realizing how much pain you were carrying without noticing. Clarity can be uncomfortable.

Theo Von

I was in so much pain. I was just trying to numb it with the alcohol. I had to address the demons within that I was trying to quiet by getting high and drunk. That's where the drugs came from, and the alcohol, just trying to self-medicate to put a smile on my face.

Mary J Blige

Being sober is my biggest act of self-love. I was like, I cannot live like this anymore, I do not want to live like this anymore. I was meant to be sober, man. I had done my time.

Travis Barker

I drank too much and it made me really unhappy. I had a problem, which is why I stopped. The difference between living life when you're drinking all the time and when you're not is really profound. It alters everything about you because you become much more part of the world. Drinking is a very self-centered way of being. You're really, really inside yourself somehow and you're not able to look out and empathize properly with people.

Ewan McGregor

I don't like the feeling of not knowing exactly what's going on at every second. I never had a cigarette and I've never had a glass of alcohol. I don't need alcohol to be happy for one second.

Gary Vaynerchuk

When I stopped drinking there were so many things I had to face that I didn't even realize were part of my makeup before. I think a lot of people are scared, and I know I was scared to get sober, at least using this as an excuse; 'I don't want to be one of those sober people.' It was a major change, and it was terrifying, but the farther you get into the woods, the less scary the woods appear. And the more time I spent working on what had caused me to be a drunk in the first place, the less afraid I was of that particular ghost returning. And as time went on, it went from being a frightening experience to being an enlightening experience. But, you know, at the time it was like losing a friend.

Jason Isbell

One day, cooped up in my hotel room, a long way from home, with nothing to think about but my own pain and misery, I suddenly knew that I had to go back into treatment. I thought to myself, 'This has got to stop.' In the lowest moments of my life, the only reason I didn't commit suicide was that I knew I wouldn't be able to drink any more if I was dead

Eric Clapton

Alcohol ate a hole in me where loving and caring had been. But all of that came back. There's life after addiction and it's good.

Joe Walsh

I've never liked the way I felt. I've had great success in my life, but I've never felt great about myself. And so, from a very early age, I used all kinds of things, anything to get me out of my head.

Ozzy Osbourne

One day, after twenty years sober, I walked into a store, saw a little bottle of Jack Daniel's, and that's how the relapse started. It's just literally being afraid. And you think, oh, this will ease the fear. And it doesn't. I was in a small town in Alaska where it's not the edge of the world, but you can see it from there, and then I thought: hey, maybe drinking will help. Because I felt alone and afraid. It was that thing of working so much, and going fuck, maybe that will help. That voice — I call it the 'lower power' — goes, "Hey. Just a taste. Just one." You feel warm and kind of wonderful. And then the next thing you know, it's a problem, and you're isolated. And it was the worst thing in the world.

Robin Williams

Alcoholics want to drink for the sole purpose of feeling better. Then the obsession of my mind kicks in. I can't stop thinking about feeling better. There is a hell. Don't let anybody tell you otherwise. I've been there: it exists: end of discussion. I was a sick guy. But I happen to know that people do change and I see that every day… They get through the terrible part of addiction, the detox, and they're able to live a normal life as long as they do a certain amount of work every day. I'm an extremely grateful guy. I'm grateful to be alive, that's for sure.

Matthew Perry

A happy drunk is something of an oxymoron. I was using drinking and drugs as a safety blanket, as a way to ignore bigger issues. It was like putting a band-aid on an untreated wound. The more memorable moments, especially during the end of my downward spiral, were not happy at all. There was a lot of crying and anger and frustration. The next day was always this overwhelming sense of disappointment. It was very evident to me that this wasn't fun anymore.

Kat Von D

I didn't realize that I was an alcoholic until I realized that the alcohol was not for fun anymore. It was medicine.

Alice Cooper

Alcohol is no longer my innate response to fear, sadness, loneliness, anger, shame. I feel more in control of my emotions. More stable. More happy. More alert. More safe. I have less anxiety socially.

Ari Lennox

I didn't think I could do anything if I wasn't drunk or high, because I was scared of everything. I let it get the better of me. I remember hitting rock bottom when I was alone in the house with two bottles of wine and was going for a third, and I thought, 'Now hold up. You're in this house by yourself going for a third bottle of wine? You might have a problem.'

Kelly Osbourne

I wouldn't turn to some sort of substance to make me feel better, I'd turn to writing. Maybe for some people drink and drugs work for them, but I'm not a tortured artist.

Mandy Moore

I had so much stuff in my life that was so good and, through abuse of drink and drugs and a continual self-flagellation, I was just fucking depressed and profoundly sad. It was miserable. In rehab they asked me again to write down what I was doing, how often I was doing it - from the first time, and when I read the list I nearly started weeping like a baby. As I was reading it, my voice caught and all of a sudden it became so sad that I or any person would have to put so much shit in their body to try and feel human or have a good time. Now I just try to remember where I was. There are still times when something's happened and I'll get down. But if I started drinking now, who knows? It would probably start slowly but I'd be fucked, fairly quickly.

Colin Farrell

Success and all that stuff doesn't make you happy. I learned that the hard way. I couldn't stop drinking. I still cannot believe that my life is what it is, because I should have died in Wales, drunk or something like that. I drank because I didn't like people. I drank because I didn't like crowds. I was a lonely man. The weird thing was happening: I was drinking more because I was more and more unhappy.

Anthony Hopkins

There was a period in my life where I was using alcohol as a self-medication. Navigating life as a woman, as a Black woman in Hollywood, is not for the faint of heart. And people cope in different ways. You don't realize how over time it gets your brain out of balance.

Sanaa Lathan

Even now, eleven years clean, I still feel the same feelings that once led me to drink and take drugs, but now I have another way to change how I feel. The priority of any addict is to numb the pain of living and ease the day with some kind of purchased relief. Whatever I endure in recovery, I need never again suffer the indignity of active addiction, the despair and hopelessness.

Russell Brand

I didn't have anything that was that important to me other than trying to dull my senses. Acting is the only thing that made me want to ever get sober. There was a time when people who didn't know me well would say, 'Couldn't you just have one glass of champagne?' And I would say, 'No.'" I've never hid it, but I've been sober the whole time I've been famous. I don't touch the stuff.

Kristin Davis

I definitely think a lot of the drinking that happened towards the end of Potter, and for a little bit after it finished. It was panic and not knowing what to do next, and not being comfortable enough in who I was to remain sober. I will always be fascinated and frustrated by the question of, "Is this something that would have happened anyway or was this to do with Potter?" Ultimately, I woke up one morning after a night going like, 'This is probably not good.'

Daniel Radcliffe

Alcoholic drinks do not agree with me. A single glass of wine or beer a day is amply sufficient to turn life into a valley of tears for me.

Friedrich Nietzsche

I went from being not particularly interested to regularly having a few pints a day before the sun had even gone down, and a shot of whiskey to go with each of them. The alcohol, though, wasn't the problem. It was the symptom. The problem was deeper. I am no longer shy of putting my hands up and saying: I'm not okay.

Tom Felton

I just feel like I'm a man. I don't feel like I need to do boyish things anymore. Maybe I'll never take another sip, who knows? My favorite vice was definitely drinking, but if I learned anything this year it's that I don't need it.

Jack Harlow

I used to think drugs and alcohol helped me cope, but they didn't, they kept me sad and super depressed. Whether I was smoking, drinking, or whatever, I wasn't liking the person that was reflecting back at me, and I was like, 'Okay, it's time to stop and sober up.

Cara Delevingne

I don't drink alcohol. Alcohol was a way I could shut my thoughts up and lose myself for hours, for days, and I didn't have to face how much

I really disliked myself. I got sober when I was 27. The reckoning came in 2014, when I realized I had to quit: 'I had to meet myself, with no one to pick up after me. I had to kind of sit with whatever chaos I caused.

Florence Welch

What is really clear is that I overdo things. And then I discovered drugs and alcohol. And that became my next chapter. I used food and drugs to numb my feelings. I was trying to quiet that voice that woke me up every morning and told me I wasn't enough. I assumed that I just didn't receive the same manual to navigate life that everyone else got at birth. I was always looking for something outside to fix my insides.

Josh Peck

When I was smashed it seemed clear I would never write songs, nor a novel, nor do much of anything, so I drank more.

Kris Kristofferson

I knew how to get wasted enough to where I took myself out of the life equation, took myself out of the present, didn't have to connect in a way that made me feel things. I had it figured out to a T but not get too drunk where I couldn't have a conversation with you. I was replacing those bottles in the bar all the time, all the time. There is a freedom that comes with not having to do those things anymore.

Jason Biggs

I've never had a drink; I've never taken a hit. One reason so many great artists die of overdoses is that they use drugs to numb pain instead of facing it. Avoiding substances gives you full access to your mind instead of numbing it. You don't need alcohol or drugs to make great art. There's never just one reason to stop drinking; there's never a real reason to keep going—only the life waiting if you stop.

Rick Rubin

Using alcohol when you are stressed or upset does not solve the problem; it just leaves you distressed and drunk at the same time. To really get sober, you need to replace the thrill of drinking with an exciting, meaningful life that can compete with alcohol. Quitting drinking is not just about stopping a habit; it is about changing how you think, act, and feel so that your future is worth staying sober for.

Jordan Petrson

Drinking was something I did to escape, but being sober has given me clarity and strength. The goal is to never again want to take anything from the outside in to feel comfortable in my present skin and that takes a lot of work. Things might be easier for me now, but my battle with addiction is a never-ending struggle.

Zac Efron

Stopping drinking has got me to a place where I'm more balanced and confident and happy and successful and a lot more proud of myself. I never had a bad relationship with alcohol, but you don't know how good life could be until you take it away.

Chris Williamson

Will I have the same amount of fun if I don't poison myself? Turns out, yes. So I think I'm done. For no reason other than it's not good for you. What kind of a moron who takes so good care of his body is poisoning himself a couple days a week for fun? When I stopped, I was like, oh my God, I feel so much better. Like, why was I poisoning myself?

Joe Rogan

When I have nothing to do I get blue and depressed, I have a natural craving for a drink. I have become convinced that there is no safety from ruin by drink except from abstaining from liquor altogether.

Ulysses S. Grant

When I got sober, I thought giving up was saying goodbye to all the fun and all the sparkle, and it turned out to be just the opposite. That's when the sparkle started for me. For me getting sober has been freedom—freedom from anxiety and freedom from…my head. We're not made to wallow in pleasure. Pleasure is joy's assassin.

Mary Karr

I'm sober 23 years. I am a solid person. I know what I think. I know what I feel. I can communicate what I think and feel. My boundaries are strong. I am a solid person today.

Jamie Lee Curtis

When you feel bad you try to escape. I tried to escape with drugs, pills and a lot of alcohol. It really destroys you.

Björn Borg

I am embarrassed how many times I quit and couldn't do it. Quit drinking and drugs. It's demoralizing. Like, I understand why people don't want to say it — because you feel like such a failure.

Dax Shepard

I quit drinking like six years ago, so I don't have the liquid courage. I just have dry courage. You have to be honest. You have to express yourself — you have to be glaringly honest... You have to express your anxieties — you can't just walk over them by drinking.

John Mayer

Alcohol became my solace. I kept thinking, 'I'll master this. I'll figure it out.' And finally, I just realized: You've never mastered this, and you never will. For my whole life, I'd felt I was weak because I wouldn't give up drinking. That inner dialogue proves to us, 'You're not capable of change. You are weak. You're staying stuck.' And when you break that cycle, the empowerment that comes out of it, that says 'I'm not weak, I'm actually strong, I've proven to myself that I am capable of change.'

Drew Barrymore

I stopped drinking and I noticed I started to sleep better, I was less anxious, and my mind wasn't racing anymore at night. There are mornings I wake up and I cannot believe that this is my life. I'm filled with gratitude. I didn't have that before.

Charlie Sheen

Food and alcohol were in my toolkit for soothing and ignoring shit that I shouldn't be soothing and ignoring. I haven't had a drink in 15 months and it's made such a huge difference in my mental health.

Valerie Bertinelli

I was filled with self-loathing and overwhelmed by shame. But I am a survivor. I've been sober for 34 years now. I've survived a lot of things. Life is full of pitfalls, even when you're sober. I can deal with them now because I don't have to run away and hide.

Elton John

I had gone from a 16-year-old who couldn't wait to grasp life to a 22-year-old who didn't care if he died in his sleep. I used to drink until I couldn't remember anything. I was just mad for it and on a death wish. It was madness. The decision to quit drinking was one of the best decisions I ever made.

Gerard Butler

I really didn't start this 'I'm never gonna drink' thing. I was like, 'I'm going on a cleanse diet', and it was like, no red meat, no bread, no alcohol. Then I did it long enough and I was like, "man, I feel amazing, why would I go back?" There's a freedom in not feeling like you need a drink to celebrate a big win or get over a tough loss. Now it's four years without drinking and working out all the time, and eating really well. To me, it's getting sober not just physically, but having emotional sobriety. It's one thing to just not drink. It's another thing to get yourself really figured out and really calm and really having emotional sobriety.

Lane Kiffin

It's been a struggle because not being able to hide behind drugs and alcohol was difficult for me. Now I deal with stuff. I'm going on 21 years sober. And that's the biggest blessing in my life

Tim Allen

I'm doing a lot better now since I stopped drinking about four months ago when my mother died. When she got sick in 2009 I started drinking every night because I couldn't sleep. I never had a problem, but I certainly was on [my] way to having one. I'd have me a nice big glass of Hennessy and I would sleep through the night. It was President Obama's visit to my studio... when he came everything became clear.

I swear the day after he left was the day I just said I am going to sleep without it.

Tyler Perry

I always drink to enhance joy. My number was 30 to 40 drinks a week. I've basically stopped and felt much better in many ways.

Amy Robach

The priority of any addict is to anesthetize the pain of living to ease the passage of day with some purchased relief. Drugs and alcohol are not my problem, reality is my problem, drugs and alcohol are my solution. But beyond today your projections of life are conceptual. You don't have to not drink for twenty years today.

Russell Brand

I was inhibited by my alcoholism and drug addiction. I used drugs and alcohol to soothe what was really a discomfort in my own skin. I would characterize the early Jackass stuff as me being palpably uncomfortable in my own skin and trying to mask that in any way I could. Over the course of time, and particularly in sobriety, I'm not masking anything. I've found my voice and my confidence.

Steve O.

I never used alcohol in any way. Covering up the emotion with pills or alcohol only allows the problem that caused the emotion to persist and get worse.

John Wooden

Drugs and alcohol were how I tried to numb grief, but I was only killing myself. The time between 1998 and 2005 was especially bad. During that time I avoided looking in the mirror, because I didn't like the person who was looking back at me. I want to lead a calm life. I'm done with partying. I don't miss alcohol in my life.

Naomi Campbell

I used to drink to quiet intense anxiety, which mostly eased when I stopped drinking. I do miss feeling loopy and carefree, but it stopped being fun toward the end. I have endless energy now, much less anxiety, and I feel more present and happier.

Chrissy Teigen

You get to a place where you feel like you are a bad person, you feel like you are a shameful person. And you feel that there's no way out, that's just who you are. Before getting sober, I would look in the mirror, call myself names, and completely despise myself. And getting sober is the process of going, 'No, I can change.' That was something I kind of clung to; the idea that I could make this huge fundamental change in who I was and how I went about my life. I'm a very, very happy, content, sober man.

Kit Harington

3. Quotes on the Mental Side

Clarity, Focus, Choices, Self-Discipline

I got tired of dragging during the day, and discovered through experimentation that even a single drink the night before was interfering with the next day. Since I stopped drinking, I feel much better. I don't need as much sleep, but my sleep is better, I'm more alert through the day, and it's easier to control my diet.

Marc Andreessen

Alcohol and sound minds do not harmonize.

Andrew Carnegie

When I think about being sober, the one word that comes to mind is clarity. Since quitting drinking, I have been grateful to wake up with a clear mind. I quit drinking in my early 20s. It has just made my life so much more simplified. I hated the feeling of being hungover and just not really having clarity. I had so much clarity in that first month of not drinking that I never drank again.

Amber Mac

I don't drink. I want to be clear-headed and focused. I grew up around alcoholics. Why would I drink?

50 Cent

There is no way anyone can perform at their best if they're dulling their brain with alcohol or drugs. I've always felt that if you want to win in anything that really matters, you need every bit of clarity and sharpness you can get, so I stay away from anything that interferes with that.

Larry Ellison

I like that I'm very lucid and clear. I don't want to live in that haze anymore. I feel alert and alive. I think the scariest addiction on this planet is to alcohol. It ruins families, it ruins relationships.

Nikki Sixx

I can't tell you how much better my life is without that shit. I mean, even if you have 5 percent more energy, 5 percent is a lot. I retain ideas longer and clearer. I wake up with ideas the way I used to.

Ben Harper

Once I was clear-headed, and I hadn't been clear-headed in so long, I was like, I can never go back. And I'm still thankful.

Travis Barker

Once I stopped drinking I found this clarity, which can be painful for a while but my life has just fallen into place.

Tom Ford

I haven't had any alcohol for a year – October 15 last year was the last time I had a drink. It has made a difference. Honestly, I think when you live cleaner, your mind is cleaner.

Jessie J

The persistent mental clarity of not drinking is amazing and life changing. It's only now that I understand the power of this.

Alex Hormozi

When you take drinking completely off the table, your mind is freed up. I'm free from all of that 'where's the next drink coming from?' stress. It has been an entirely positive experience. I'm so much happier, I can't even tell you, and everything about my life is better. You don't find anybody who regrets quitting drinking. We've been sold this lie that drinking is a happier life and sober is deprivation. And it's just not the case.

Catherine Gray

If something keeps making you do dumb things, you remove it from your life. Alcohol is on that list. When I left the SEAL Teams, I walked out of the bars. I had other things to do, and I was done with that. I just kind of stopped drinking… now I just don't drink anymore.

Jocko Willink

I'm sharper, I'm more creative, I'm more present with my family. I was so concerned what you thought of me, how I was coming across, how I would survive the day. I always felt like an outsider. I just lived in my head. I've been very lucky. I feel more myself than I have in years.

Bradley Cooper

When I turned 40, I realized even one glass of wine made me feel different the next day, so I stopped. Everyone says a little wine is healthy, but for my body it wasn't. Without alcohol I feel clearer, I sleep better, and I can show up as my best self. Alcohol made me foggy; sobriety makes me present.

Gisele Bündchen

I was never a serious drinker at all. But it was one of those conscious decisions that, you know, I wanted to be more successful. I want to remember things with more clarity. I want to be sharper. I want to be more precise. I want to be able to study. People say, you know, "Charlie, how do you remember all this stuff?" First of all, I have a good memory. I work hard at it. I eat very clean, but also I don't drink. I'm not poisoning my body. I don't mean to attack people that drink. Plenty of good people do. But it is poison. I mean, it is actual poison.

Charlie Kirk

I can honestly say, all the bad things that ever happened to me were directly, directly attributed to drugs and alcohol. I would never piss on a piece of stone at the Alamo at nine o'clock in the morning dressed in a woman's evening dress sober. I don't get in my car drunk any more.

Ozzy Osbourne

When you take a drink, your whole thinking changes immediately. And you do things that you normally wouldn't do if you were sober.

Elton John

Liquor creates delusion. It can make your life feel full of risk and adventure, sparkling and dynamic as a rough sea under sunlight. A single drink can make you feel unstoppable, masterful, capable of solving problems that overwhelmed you just five minutes before. In fact, the opposite is true: drinking brings your life to a standstill, makes it static as rock over time. When you quit drinking you stop waiting. The hard things in life, the things you really learn from, happen with a clear mind.

Caroline Knapp

All the mistakes I've ever made in my life have been when I've been drunk. I haven't made hardly any mistakes sober, ever.

Tracey Emin

Let's put it this way: I did not get in trouble every time I drank, but every time I got in trouble, I'd been drinking. Sobriety has given me everything back that alcohol took away.

Dave Mustaine

You end up losing cognitive function, memory, inhibition, self-control. You think you're getting away with it, but you're not. My cheeks would turn bright red and my speech would get slurred. It was getting to be too much. And it had got to the point where, every time I did it, it was becoming more and more debilitating.

John Goodman

A number of things made me come to the conclusion that I didn't want to drink. First and foremost, I didn't feel it had a place where I personally wanted to be. My mental and physical health became a lot more important to me than feeling like I had to be 'on' at a party or social setting. I'm not going to lie... the fact that I looked better because I wasn't drinking was also incentive to not veer from the road I am on. The truth is I don't miss it at all. All I know is I have never felt better physically or been more clear mentally.

Kyle Richards

They say the day you start drinking is actually the day you stop maturing, and then when you get sober, you start at that age and then move through that. I'm actually not 50, I'm only 29. Addiction robbed me of 21 years of maturity.

Theo Fleury

When I was drinking, I mean, I really felt like I couldn't cope with my life. I felt like it was all too hard. Alcohol is a deceptive drug. It creates the illusion of pleasure and relaxation while causing the very anxiety and discomfort it purports to relieve. Even for the lighter or more occasional drinker who has decided to stop, they very soon forget the vast majority of drinks that they took that did nothing for them, and remember the few here and there that they really enjoyed.

William Porter

I didn't want to quit – the idea terrified me! Wine was my best friend. I really believed alcohol brought out the best in me, that I needed it to be confident and fun. Alcohol and I had been together for over twenty years. We'd had some great times, but recently it had been making me feel depressed, fat, and ill. It was time we split up.

Clare Pooley

I was using wine to decompress, to ease into the second shift of the evening — and so too were my friends. Wine was my consolation, my friend at the end of the day, my companion in crime. A drink is a punctuation mark of sorts, between day and night.

Ann Dowsett Johnston

I didn't think I had a problem with alcohol. I thought, 'I didn't drink every day, so I don't have a problem.' It wasn't how often I drank, it was what I did when I drank that was the problem. I had to change my thoughts. At the core, it wasn't just the alcohol or the pills, it was the way I thought. I was in rehab for 28 days, and it worked. While I was there I admitted that I had a serious problem, and I did everything I could to tackle each and every one of my underlying issues. When I got out, the toughest thing was the first three months, because I had to change my thought process.

Brett Favre

It starts off as a fun little thing, then it turns into an escape. If something bad happens you drink in an attempt to forget; if something good happens you drink in order to celebrate; and if nothing happens you drink to make something happen.

James Hetfield

When I first got sober, I never thought I'd be funny again. I never thought I could play guitar in front of people without a buzz. And one day at a time, you learn how to do it. Getting sober was the hardest thing I've ever had to do. Because alcohol had convinced me that I couldn't do anything without it.

Joe Walsh

Now I feel free. I don't drink. I don't take pills. Nothing. And it's fantastic. It's like getting out of prison.

Melanie Griffith

As much as I loved football, there was something else in college and high school that I got really good at, and that was partying. As things started to go bad in my football life, I turned to something else that I was really good at. Where did that get me except out of the NFL?

Johnny Manziel

I know it's not easy to get sober. I've been there. It was tough to come to that decision. But I made the choice, and I came out stronger. It's made my life exponentially better — just more sharp, more focused, clearer thinking... and then for sure on the athletic side with what it does to your body.

Jake Paul

I tried to moderate every time I drank, but I couldn't. I decided that I didn't want to moderate; I wanted to quit drinking altogether. In quitting, I learned how to be the person I wanted to be. The first year was 365 days of inner turmoil as I tried to learn a new way of life, to cope, and to function. In quitting, I didn't lose anything. I gained everything.

Celeste Yvonne

I used the excuse that I needed to do this because it was fueling my art. I wasted a lot of time. I romanticized the idea of alcohol. Every day we weren't playing I'd be in the hotel room trying not to be sick, and it sucked. I wound up in a very bad place. I got sober, and it really kind of turned my brain back on. Getting sober just exploded my life. Now I have a much clearer sense of myself and what I want to do. Once I got on stable ground and started to understand how my brain worked without all that, I can do more because I can remember what I did. I can think deeper about things.

Trent Reznor

The real reason I stopped drinking, though, was because I decided that I had had enough. That moment came for me one morning when I woke up on the floor of my apartment after a particularly out of control night. I didn't know what the alternative to drinking was at this point. I didn't know what was going to come next, I just knew that I didn't want this anymore.

Hayley Gibson

When my pals in high school were starting to drink, it always looked unappealing to me. I would be at a big party and see one of the popular girls or football players completely wasted and puking and acting a fool, and think to myself, 'There's nothing cool about that. I never wanted to be that out of control.

Kathy Griffin

After a while, when you wake up in the morning, you wake up feeling, 'Who do I owe a phone call to? Who do I need to apologize to? Why am I covered in bruises? Who is that?' I have a problem with moderation, where every night would lead to a blackout. I used to wake up in unfamiliar places with no memory of how I got there. My life is much better without it.

Janeane Garofalo

My decision to quit alcohol for a year came after I realized it was controlling me rather than I controlling it. I decided to take a break, so I could retrain my brain and the relationship it has formed with alcohol over the years. I did a lot of reading on habits and alcohol and spent a fair bit of time looking inwards and thinking about why I drank and what was behind it. Having a break from alcohol was one of the best things I've ever done.

Sarah Jane Clarke

Elite athletes aren't easy people to get sober. We have pretty big egos, usually. I was not a bad person, but under the influence, I was making a lot of bad decisions and doing bad things. I'd become everything that I hated in life, and I didn't even see it coming. I didn't love or respect myself, but today I do. There's not a part of my life that sobriety hasn't changed.

Carrie Bates

When I had my first drink in high school, I was like, 'This is the answer to all my problems.' By college, I knew I had a drinking problem. I just could not stop drinking. Alcohol is cunning, baffling—the disease of addiction is cunning, baffling, and powerful. I would try to stop drinking, and I couldn't. I tried so many times to get sober on my own for eight years in a row. I'd get three years and three months and I'd go back to drinking. I'd get a year in recovery, or being sober, and I'd go back to drinking.

Kathryn Burgum

Three years alcohol free today. When I look back, I barely recognize the person I was. My drinking was completely out of control. My anxiety was paralyzing. I hated who I became when I drank and I felt completely lost. Sobriety has been the ultimate act of self-love. It has been messy and hard and uncomfortable at times but it has transformed me in ways I never thought possible.

Millie Mackintosh

Alcohol was my comfort blanket. I made the decision for many personal reasons for myself where I knew enough was enough and I had to take total control of that. Alcohol was the biggest plaster I could put on myself. The fake me has completely gone and I don't ever want to have that back. It's precious to me, REALLY precious, to have the clarity. I went completely cold turkey. If you'd told me I would toast my 40th birthday with a glass of water, I'd have thought you were crackers.

Lisa Riley

I feel like I've grown up. I don't want to be that person who's out all night anymore. I was not very happy. I was doing things that weren't good for me. People aren't themselves when they drink, and they say things that they would never say when they were sober.

Kate Moss

I was trying to drink myself into being someone else. I'd drink so much that I'd wake up with no idea what I'd done the night before. That scared me. I had to learn to live life on life's terms without picking up a drink. That's therapy too, when you take responsibility for all the foolishness you're doing. You got to feel it, deal, then heal.

Mary J. Blige

At one time I was definitely on the verge of alcoholism. I would be on the floor in the toilets, crying, having panic attacks, and unable to perform. I would drink before going on stage, I thought it would calm my nerves, but it actually made things so much worse. I knew that if I carried on drinking the way I was, I would just completely lose control of my life.

Ellie Goulding

I don't feel the need to drink because I know how it will affect me at 3 in the morning when I wake up with horrible anxiety thinking about that one thing I said five years ago when I graduated high school.

Bella Hadid

People that have only known me since sobriety, they'll be like, 'I can't imagine what you're like when you were drunk.' And I'm always like, 'I was fucking horrible. I would turn into kind of a bully. When I was drinking, I could be quite mean. It would be fun for a minute, but then it would go to quite a dark place.

Lily Allen

Ultrarunners can't be alcoholics, can they? I managed to convince myself that all the running meant that my drinking was okay; because I was exercising, I could drink more. Drinking is great because you can always blame it. Your behavior can be horrendous and then you say, 'It was just because I was pissed,' and everyone lets you off. If you are asking yourself if you have a troubled relationship with alcohol, you have a troubled relationship with alcohol. When I got sober, I had to do a lot of work on myself.

Allie Bailey

I couldn't just have one or two. I had to have ten. My off switch was broken. I had to lose everything—my marriage, my money, and my self-respect—before I was willing to change. I was a world-record holder by day and a blackout drunk by night. One of the things I love about sobriety is that you have that clarity, that accountability. When you're a drunk, you can blame everybody and everything but yourself.

Karlyn Pipes

Calling myself sober, and not ingesting ethanol on the regular, led to greater clarity, and also a mad desire to break through all the limitations I had accepted for my life. Quitting drinking was also where the jig of treating myself like shit was up. I had no choice but to accept that I alone was responsible for taking care of this precious person whose life I was charged with.

Holly Whitaker

When I first got sober, my biggest reservation was that I was terrified of becoming boring. Once I removed the substances, I was able to see how incredibly unpredictable, how incredibly un-boring, life can be.

Cat Marnell

It's strange. Nobody starts out to be a drunk. It's the 'creeping disease. You never start out in life with the intention of becoming a bankrupt or an alcoholic or a cheat and a thief. Or a liar. It finally dawned on me that I couldn't drink like a normal person. I suppose I wanted to live. It's very painful to think about some of the things that happened back then. I made a wasteland out of everything I touched.

Raymond Carver

Why couldn't I stop after 6 or 7 drinks? Why didn't I have an 'off' switch when I had that first drink every day? Well, 'Why?' is not a useful question. I decided that the single most subversive, revolutionary thing I could do was to show up for my life and not be ashamed.

Anne Lamott

I was thinking about booze all the time. Somebody once asked me how I define sobriety, and my response was 'liberation from dependence.'

Leslie Jamison

I suppose I lucked out in that I don't really like the taste of alcohol, and it just puts me to sleep. I was never into drugs or alcohol. That was fortunate. I don't have a propensity to be addicted to those things. It was never my thing. My brain tires.

Andrew Huberman

The blackouts were horrible. It was hideous to let those nights slide into a crack in the ground. You drink so much that your long-term memory shuts down. So you're still walking and talking and interacting with people, but the recorder in your brain isn't going.

Sarah Hepola

I'm a good teacher. My affection for my students is what keeps me tethered to reality. I lose that connection every day after school when I drive away from the parking lot towards the grocery store to grab two large bottles of wine. It doesn't seem like being alive is as hard for other people as it is for me. It just feels like there's some kind of secret to life I don't know.

Glennon Doyle

I don't drink alcohol. Drinking alcohol is a terrible way for you to moderate your negative affect because all you'll get is more negative affect tomorrow. The pursuit of pleasure does not lead to happiness; instead, it results in addiction. You're going to hit the button, and hit the button, and you're going to become miserable, doing that until you break free.

Arthur Brooks

To stop drinking, all you have to do is sit. In 100 percent of the documented cases of alcoholism worldwide, the people who recovered all shared one thing in common: They didn't drink. If I was going to be completely sober for the rest of my life, then the life I lived needed to be a life from which I did not seek escape. I've been sober since 1999. To stop drinking, all you have to do is sit. Do you want to be sober more than you want to drink? You have to replace alcohol with something else. You have to replace it. I had no idea how to fill the day when I got sober. Writing about it at least gave me something to do with my hands.

Augusten Burroughs

I woke up with one of the worst vulnerability hangovers of my life. You know that feeling when you wake up and everything feels fine until the memory of laying yourself open washes over you and you want to hide under the covers? What did I do?

Brené Brown

All the time I was drinking I thought I was doing it to find myself and now I know it was keeping me from myself. My recovery started the second I was able to not just admit that I had a problem, but actually talk about it with the people around me, and to be brutally honest and not lie about how many drinks I had.

Abby Wambach

Addiction can have me thinking all kinds of crazy things. Recovery isn't just not using. It's changing the way you think, the way you move, the way you show up for people. It's not the using that's the battle. It's your thinking—your self-centeredness at the center of it all. And if you still suffer from that thinking, you'll pick up something else to be addicted to.

Darren Waller

It took me 28 years to realize that I had a problem. The planning out of it, what made me realize I was an alcoholic, I was planning out when I could drink. If you've got to do that, I feel like you've got a problem. When I'm coming out of the game, I needed a Crown and Sprite in my locker. So I would literally start after the last pitch I threw. If I pitched on a Monday, I would be intoxicated by Tuesday through Wednesday, detoxing with just water and Gatorade on Thursday and Friday. By Saturday, I'd be ready for a Crown and Sprite at my locker after the game. I never really wanted to stop drinking. The hardest part is actually facing it and telling somebody you need help.

CC Sabathia

You can't start treating something until you know what you have, until you admit that you have it. Labeling myself as an alcoholic was one of the best things I had ever done, as opposed to just pretending like everything was okay. Everybody has issues that they have to deal with — some physical, some mental.

Steve Sarkisian

Do I feel ashamed by some of the choices I made? Hell yeah. They were despicable. I was basically just committing suicide. When you're an addict, nothing can get through to you. I never thought I was going to die. I never thought I'd be in a coma. I didn't think I had a problem. But then I woke up in a bed with tubes coming out of my mouth — and it was real.

Lamar Odom

I don't drink anymore. There is no room for late night binges, spontaneous cheat days or emotional eating. What you eat and drink affects your temperament, focus, confidence, and sleep.

Virat Kohli

I had many moments and many nights when I would wake up and I won't remember what the hell just happened that night. It was years of waking up in the middle of the night, unable to remember how I got home, walking downstairs and cracking the garage door open to see if my car was there.

Sugar Ray Leonard

Even if I stopped running, I'll not go to drinking. It's not in my mentality. I trust that if you drink you forget something and I don't want to forget; I want to live a life where the young generation can see the positive parts. Self-discipline can help you to actually get three things. It can save your feelings. Get you back on the course when you try to think otherwise, self-discipline can help easily come back and think positively. It helps you do the right thing in the moment for long-term benefits

Eliud Kipchoge

If I think I can have one drink, I think I can have two, and then it snowballs to 10 or 12. Any time I drink, there's a point that comes where a switch flips and you never know when that point's going to be reached, whether it's the first three or four, or the 15th. And that's what's so dangerous about it. Addiction is a humbling experience. Getting it under control is even more humbling.

Josh Hamilton

My problem has always not just been when things are bad I turn to drugs and alcohol, but when things are good I turn to drugs and alcohol. People say, 'Don't do drugs, just drink.' Alcohol is a drug. And I know if I do one I'm going to do the other I Any time I would feel bad or feel good, that was like my scapegoat. There were times I would literally be crying going to buy drugs or going to a liquor store.

Doc Gooden

Two, three pints I'm gone, especially beer. I'm senseless, speechless drunk. Especially if you don't drink all of the time. I tried drinking and it's not for me – I get pissed after four pints.

Tyson Fury

When I first had that first drink, I was like, 'Oh my God, this is like my savior.' But over time, I noticed all the bad decisions I was making in my life all revolved around drinking. I was getting into trouble, I wasn't being a professional. Sobriety saved my life.

Maxx Crosby

Partying was, I felt, a defining feature of my personality. But hedonism was like a disguise. I was a shy kid and had to alter my personality. At first it's freeing, but then it becomes a prison of its own making. Once I drank, the alcohol would just tell me what to do, or who I was hanging out with, or whatever, and I had no real independence with it. It sort of ruled my whole life.

Florence Welch

For 12 years I was drinking, and for 11 and a half I didn't want to stop. Alcohol is an unbelievable drug. The denial was really strong. I've got no angst of the past anymore. I've cleaned that up – I'm 28 years without a drink or a drug. I'm comfortable in my own skin for the first time in my life.

Tony Adams

I just kept getting in trouble, fucking up, being unhealthy. I wasn't having any fun with it at all anymore. It was just a drag, the whole thing. Quitting drinking was very gradual. It's not that much fun anymore anyway. With drugs and drink you're always chasing some memory of having a really good time which is hard to recreate.

Slash

My life is so much better since I stopped living in a haze. People romanticize it, and even I romanticized it. When I was drinking, I was working and I was remembering lines, so you feel you're getting away with it, though, deep down, beneath the denial, you know. I said to myself, 'I cannot live like this anymore. I do not want to live like this anymore.'

Gary Oldman

There was a period of six years, from 16 to 21, when I was a bit of a party animal. I've been sober since my early twenties. I made a choice, because drinking wasn't a good addition to my life. I immediately felt a change when I quit drinking. Some kids really mess up their lives. They get too involved with alcohol and drugs. Other kids try it and then get out of it really quickly. Other kids just don't even go near it, and I think they're the ones that are better off.

Christina Ricci

I thought I could handle my alcohol, but I didn't realize how much your body and your life changes when it's not in your life every day. It's nice to wake up with clarity. I'm glad to be done with it. It is worth being a present, non-hungover person. It's also nice to be super sober for sex.

Chelsea Handler

I would drink until I couldn't remember anything. I was a textbook binge drinker, blacking out. I wouldn't remember what I did or what I said, which was scary. When I got sober, my intention was never to be the poster child of sobriety. When I began speaking about it, it came from a place of needing to heal and take my power back. And I can't believe I'm now at a place in my life where I can talk about the things that used to bring me so much shame. I love that I am just showing up as myself and not having to paint a pretty picture of what people expect me to be or expect me to say. Where my life is at now is just trying to be as present as possible.

Lucy Hale

I don't think I'll ever drink again. It was leading me to be in all these situations, you know, waking up in the morning being like, Who did I meet last night? What did I say? I liked being drunk; I just hated the hangover where I regretted what had happened.

Nikki Glaser

Alcohol is universally presented as the fast track to fun, relaxation, celebration, and joy. But I knew that I felt so much better without it. I was a problem drinker. My problem drinking just didn't look like what I thought problem drinking was. For many of us, it begins with a simple question: Would my life be better without alcohol?" To discover the answer for yourself, all that remains is to put the cork back in the bottle, open your eyes, and see.

Ruby Warrington

After my accident honestly didn't want to put anything in my body when I got out. Once I was clear-headed, and I hadn't been clear-headed in so long, I was like, I can never go back. And I'm still thankful.

Travis Barker

I really do believe in the connection of your bodily health to your mental health, so staying healthy and taking time to do a stress-relieving activity every day. Someone said, 'You quit drinking? You're not even 21 yet,' and I was like, 'I crammed a lot into a few years.' It's not the kind of life that I want to live or the kind of thing I think is fun or attractive.

Julien Baker

When I got sober, I was able to pay attention to the world more, and awareness is the most important tool for any creative person. I know now what was really scaring me was just the thought of getting sober. At the time, I thought it was: "Am I going to be funny?...Are people going to be attracted to me anymore?...Am I going to be interesting?" What's going to happen to this romantic sort of Hemingway idea I have of my life? But all those things were bullshit. That was the addiction wanting to continue and wanting to feed itself and keep itself alive. I look back on it and I realize that I was never interesting because I was drunk. That was not why people were hanging out with me. And I wasn't fun because I was drunk. And I'm certainly more attractive than I was then in every conceivable way. But the addiction in your brain, that's a tricky son of a bitch. It had me convinced for a long time that I wasn't going to enjoy my life, that nobody was going to enjoy being around me if I wasn't raising hell all the time.

Jason Isbell

I don't miss alcohol in my life. I feel better without it. I felt a bit more foggy before. Now I'm very sharp and very present, and I notice things that I didn't notice before. With every sober day, I remember who I was before alcohol.

Naomi Campbell

What makes me an alcoholic is not how much I drank or how often I used. it's what happens to me and who I become when I do, and I don't like that guy. Getting clean was the hardest — and best — thing I've ever done.

Steven Tyler

Right up until the time I stopped drinking, everything I said was complete blather. The noise in my head was deafening, and drinking was in my thoughts all the time. I'd reached the point where I couldn't live without a drink and I couldn't live with one. I was a mess. Staying sober really was the most important thing in my life. It gave me direction when I thought I had none.

Eric Clapton

I was drinking daily and partying a lot. When I stopped, I gained a lot of clarity into what I was capable of accomplishing when my head was sober and focused on the greater good.

Soko

When I got arrested, I was very sick and I was in the process of losing everything that was dear to me. I had not played a show for two years and was out of communication with the guys in Phish. I was very sick and skinny and crazy and mean. It hurts my head to talk about this stuff, but it's true. I think the trickiest part was that I didn't understand how deep in it I had gone. You're kind of a crazy person at that point in time. You are. And I was almost like an alien in my own landscape. It's taken years—and it will probably be a lifetime—of unravelling how far I had strayed from my inner compass.

Trey Anastasio

I've been sober for 25 years. My sobriety lets me see all the lightness and darkness in me more clearly. You have to be present enough to understand when it's time to give certain things up, but you also need tools to know how to deal with being present.

RuPaul

If you need booze or drugs to enjoy your life to the fullest you are doing it wrong. Most of the time you just realize you've started to do embarrassing things. There is this thing for alcoholics called a black out which isn't really a black out it's more like sleepwalking with activities. I was shameful, and you do stuff that causes disgust. As an alcoholic, you will violate your standards quicker than you can lower them.

Robin Williams

It's nice to be present. Sobriety is a very present experience. It's nice to remember events as they are happening.

Ari Lennox

I was at a dinner party about year into my sobriety and everyone was drinking but me. Someone at the table insulted me quite out of nowhere—like, she kind of stabbed me right in the guts with her words, and right in front of everyone. It hurt, yes, and definitely took me by surprise because it seemed to come out of nowhere. But because I was sober, I was able to clock how alcohol had changed this person's personality throughout the night, and how she was glassy-eyed and slurring. I was able to see how she wasn't really THERE, how this wasn't really HER speaking, but the booze. I could see how out of control she was, and how ashamed and shook she herself seemed to feel about what she had said.

Maybe the insult was, in fact, her true opinion about me, or maybe it wasn't—I'll never know. But I knew for sure that she would never have said those words six drinks earlier in the evening.

Seeing her recklessness and subsequent shame made me feel so grateful that I was not six drinks in, myself. And I knew that if I'd had any mind-altering substances coursing through my body when the insult was launched, I wouldn't have been able to be calm, detached, and clear-headed about having been insulted.

That was maybe the first night when I saw what a superpower sobriety is—how it allowed me to stand a bit of a safe remove from the human drama and messiness that was going on at the table, and to not have to be pulled into every bit of chaos that was happening around me. It felt kind of amazing, to be able to hold my serenity in such a moment. I remember thinking that night, "I never want my perspective be clouded or diminished by anything again."

Elizabeth Gilbert

I gave up drinking because bad things happened. Things that you just think, 'I really shouldn't have done that.' There have been lots of gigs where I've looked back and gone, 'Oh, it was on television, a lot of people saw that, and I was totally inebriated.'

Calvin Harris

I used to drink too much, and then I would black out and I would 'ruin' parties, or so I'm told. When you do that enough — when you black out drinking and you do crazy things — you kind of become like Michael Jackson, like any story anyone says about you might be true, and even you don't know by the end. I drank too much and I had to stop.

John Mulaney

I've never been drunk in my life. Nothing. I have an addictive personality... so me being aware of that — if I ended up liking alcohol or some shit — that would be the fucking downfall of me.

Tyler the Creator

Later on, towards the middle of my life, I grew more and more opposed to alcoholic drinks... The peoples are so greatly deceived because they are always seeking a deceiver: that is to say, a wine to stimulate their senses.

Friedrich Nietzsche

Upon reflection with friends and family this weekend, I have come to the conclusion that I will be a better person without alcohol in my life. My problems with alcohol are not an excuse for my personal lapses in judgment. I stopped because I thought it was a good thing to stop.

Gavin Newsom

I've seen that drunk people know about the future, but they don't care about it. I grew up in a very hard drinking culture, drank heavily into my twenties, and finally decided at 27 that I had had enough. Alcohol temporarily lifts the terrible burden of self-consciousness. To continue the warm glow, the drinker may just continue to drink. They can party like there's no tomorrow. But because there is a tomorrow, drunk people also get in trouble.

Jordan Peterson

The increased mental sharpness was something I really didn't expect because I already thought I was relatively sharp. But over time I found that my memory and my verbal agility and my creativity had all improved far more than I thought they would. This kicked in really hard after about three months, and it felt like a brain fog had been lifted.

Chris Williamson

Alcohol ruined me financially and morally, broke my heart and the hearts of too many others. Even though it did this to me and it almost killed me and I haven't touched a drop of it in seventeen years, sometimes I wonder if I could get away with drinking some now. I totally subscribe to the notion that alcoholism is a mental illness because thinking like that is clearly insane.

Craig Ferguson

When I had alcohol in me I did things I'd never do sober.

Dax Shepard

You have to fight really hard to look at it from a critical point of view because it's constantly pushed on you. Every Friday and Saturday, on social media, there is enabling going on for drinking. I just tapped out. The quality of life has gone up considerably. Drinking is a fucking con. How much is enough? Every time I drank, I was looking for some sort of regulated amount. "I said two, now it's three, now we're at four?"

John Mayer

I started regretting some things I did when I was drunk. It's funny to be obnoxious or out of control, but then it's like, 'I think I hurt that person's feelings, I made a fool of myself, or I didn't want to kiss that girl.' I have almost no inhibitions, so it's dangerous for me. I just wanted to stop.

Ben Affleck

So, I had a major surgery. I had my hip replaced and I said, "I'm just going to try it [abstinence]after the surgery. And I just felt better and better and I felt quicker. Yes. I think the most important thing is that I was able to, like when I had struggles, I was able to recover from them quicker.

Colin Plume

I always think about the downtimes, how it made me feel, and how I fouled up everything I ever did in my life. Everything I did that was screwy had some alcohol in it. I'm a slow learner, but by God, I've learned.

Joe Namath

Even with life struggles and how life can be challenging, I find that it is easier to get myself clearer faster, about what I need to do and taking care of my life. I feel good when I wake up in the morning. I'm not groggy. I'm not tired. I'm not: 'What did I do last night?'"

Valerie Bertinelli

I was kind of turning into a party boy at night. That resulted in me getting fired and that was enough to crumble me. I needed to learn a hard lesson and grow up. I was using alcohol to like just check out, so I didn't have to deal with the problems. I was worried about the wrong stuff and trying to chase things that didn't matter. I had to learn what I could control and what I couldn't, and picking up a drink is something I can absolutely control.

Mike McDanile

Sobriety is, like, that's like my God. I need it, I live for it. It's changed my entire life.

Miley Cyrus

My dad was a bad alcoholic, so I haven't had a drink in 45 years. I saw what it did to him and said, 'I just don't ever want to go there'.

Dr. Phil McGraw

Drinking to escape was profoundly selfish. I was self-medicating. I was in denial because I thought, I can't be an alcoholic. I'm not homeless, I'm not jobless, I'm a mother, I'm a wife, I'm a network news anchor. I'm all these things. Therefore I cannot be an alcoholic.

Elizabeth Vargas

My goal was to go my entire life without ever drinking alcohol. I've drank like five times in my life; I don't like the way it makes me feel. It just makes me feel stupid, but not a good stupid. It's not like a happy stupid. So I don't drink alcohol. For decades, I've chosen work over nights out.

MrBeast (Jimmy Donaldson)

I didn't love myself. I didn't respect my own power. Today I do. I own my personal power with soulful courage. I am wildly honest and comfortably open. I am free. I needed to stop drinking alcohol because it kept my mind and heart circling in the same direction. I had so much self-discovery to unlock and explore.

Jessica Simpson

When I stopped drinking, my own friends started questioning who I was. I knew several people who felt threatened by my decision because they weren't ready to face their own relationship with alcohol. Your friends could be struggling, even when they're posting these beautiful lifestyle pictures. But are you aware? Because it is socially acceptable, the addiction side of it, the bad sides of it, really do fly under the radar. I don't drink alcohol and many people are often confused or wonder why. Short answer: because I love my BRAIN!

Jay Shetty

I'm not a drinker. I want nothing to interfere with my own thought process.

David Goggins

I used to drink a lot. That was a hard time in my life. I would drink every day. I would drink alone. I thought the whole concept was so fucking cool. At first it's fine and you think you have a dark side – it's exciting – and then you realize the dark side wins every time if you decide to indulge it. I knew it was a problem when I liked it more than I liked doing anything else. It's been many years since my last drink.

Lana Del Rey

4. Quotes on the Social Side

Popularity, Fun, Inhibitions, Peer Pressure

I think we just live in a culture where it's like you're the weird one if you're not drinking, which is like crazy because it's this thing that's poisoning you and can create a lot of problems and distract you from working hard in life. People think you're lame if you're not drinking, but honestly, it's the opposite… you're the one actually in control.

Jake Paul

My big worry when I got sober was I wasn't going to have fun anymore. I was young. I was 26. I was like I'm not giving up my fun. But I have more fun today than I ever had in the days when I was drinking and drugging and doing all this stuff. Being sober can be so much fun.

Rob Lowe

There's this whole belief that you can only have fun with alcohol. I had to really reprogram that aspect, because it's just all over in our culture. So, I haven't missed it. My life has definitely become more of a morning life, but I can still go out and have fun.

Sanaa Lathan

I wanted to be that girl. The girl who could have a glass of wine at dinner, or do a tequila shot at a party. So I tried to become that: a fun, normal girl. I opened that door to drinking after almost 20 years of sobriety. I wanted to be something other than who I am. And I gave my power away.

Demi Moore

I didn't learn until I stopped drinking that people actually like me better when I don't drink. All of a sudden my product as a human being, as a husband, as a coach, was a completely better product and something that I think those lessons really, in that time in my life, sealed the deal for me.

Mike McDaniel

It's really hard because, especially being young, there's that stigma of 'You're no fun'. It's like, 'Honey, you can call me a lot of things, but I know that I'm fun.' I don't think that everyone has to be sober. Everyone has to do what's best for them. I don't have a problem with drinking, I have a problem with the decisions I make once I go past a certain level.

Miley Cyrus

With much thought, I eventually realized I was drinking alcohol to survive longer in social environments which I wasn't particularly happy in. I now have a rule: only associate with people where you don't have to drink to be around them.

Naval Ravikant

Why do I sometimes feel like an outsider if I say I don't drink? Growing up in a society where we have what I call a 'dominant drinking culture,' whether or not we become a drinker often does not feel like a choice. I really started to question this, and the more I began to pull out of what I've come to terms the dominant drinking culture, the more clarity I began to get around the way I was using alcohol. I realized how much alcohol played a role in my relationships so I cut it out and have never felt happier.

Ruby Warrington

Alcohol is the only drug on earth you have to justify NOT taking. I have been the lone sober person at many of these occasions. Here's what happens. The wine comes, and the mood changes, so the conversation is intelligent, quick-witted, and full of life. Fast forward two or three glasses, and conversation grows a bit dull, even among some of the most intelligent people. The wine does exactly what it is supposed to; it slows your brain function and dulls your senses.

Annie Grace

If I'm at a party, as soon as that wave of everybody being drunk starts, I'm out of there. I don't drink, and I cannot be around drunk people. I'd have to be honest: I have contempt for pretty much every drug other than pot. I find drunk people gross.

Sarah Silverman

I hated going into bars and being with drunks. But I loved the music and so I survived. I'm not one of those people who stays up until four in the morning eating pizza and drinking beer. I don't drink. I don't do drugs. And I eat well. I like to stay fit. I like a clean band. I like to have clean-living people around me.

Shania Twain

There is a pressure within a social setting. You have that one shot and are like, 'Damn, why did I do that?' when you get home. I always felt awkward in those settings. I was like, wow that's kind of crazy how I'm feeling pressured. And I realized, how can I be feeling pressure at 38?.

Lewis Hamilton

I would get really uncomfortable and not confident in social scenarios out in public. That's why I really latched onto drinking because it masked that insecurity with stupidity. I used to go to these parties, and be like, "I can't speak to someone until I'm drunk."

Tom Holland

Wine was my best friend. I was the party girl, the rebel. Wine defined me. So, I tried, and tried to moderate. I thought I'd be giving up fun, spontaneity, holidays, parties. Instead, I gave up hangovers, 3 a.m. shame, and the constant anxiety about how much I'd drunk. The more I tried to drink less, the more I thought about booze. Moderation just isn't my thing. I quit drinking on 2nd March 2015. Going sober has transformed my life.

Clare Pooley

Sober people are not boring. I find some of the most interesting, complex, beautiful human beings that I know struggle in this way.

Lucy Hale

I turned to alcohol as a social lubricant. That helped me at the time until it stopped helping me. I got sober at 25 because I didn't want to die. And because I really believed there had to be something more than what I was doing. I haven't had a drink or a drug since.

Amber Valletta

I was very shy — with strangers — I couldn't talk to people. And I found if I had a drink, it would loosen me up. The barriers went down, and I became very social. That's what got me started. It took me a long time to get over it. I get a lot of letters from people who say all of a sudden they weren't ashamed to admit they had a drinking problem and they got help. So, I'm very proud of that.

Dick Van Dyke

Your friend group changes when you get sober. The first thing that happens is your real friends emerge. All the people who loved you, who you were probably hurting when you were drinking, and who had disappeared and were infuriating you and fighting with you, it turns out they were fighting with you because they loved you and they were worried. My wife, Sue, my parents, the three band members in Phish, and my band members in my solo band, and a couple of friends from high school were right there. Ninety percent of the people I was hanging out with just vanished. Boom—they were gone. The party moved on. And now I'm clean and sober. My children are happy. In August, my wife and I will celebrate our fifteenth wedding anniversary. My band is back together with a sold-out tour. Drinking and drugging, for me it was a slow death of isolation.

Trey Anastasio

I don't drink because I don't like the effects of alcohol, but I like being a part of it. I like being social. I like people coming together. I found that sometimes not drinking, the thing that was interesting was that it was a little alienating, because you don't feel — and maybe it's just in your own head — but you just don't really feel a part of it.

Blake Lively

I can totally party. If I decide to go out, I can be out till 6 a.m. and be sober and be completely fine. But it needs to be the right time and the right place and the right people. I think there's something that most people find quite charismatic about people that are like carefree and live that way, but I see so past that. I'm like, "I'm really sorry that you're in pain, and I'm really sorry that you need a crutch, and I'm really sorry that this is your way to tune out from the world.

Soko

I'm not really an 'alcohol girl' There's this whole belief that you can only have fun with alcohol. I had to really reprogram that aspect, because it's just all over in our culture. It's not like I decided on these strict lifestyle choices and I'm enforcing them. It's just something that I genuinely don't have a desire for. I feel like I've been very lucky because I don't really have an addictive personality. I've never had any drugs, and I had a little taste of alcohol when I was 12 years old, but that's about it.

Tyra Banks

When I stopped it was like, 'Wow, you know, I used to tell myself that it was a social thing, but after a year and a half without it I became very social. After two years I was like, why did I wait so long to stop? I'm more social now than I've been ever in my life.'

Janeane Garofalo

It's scary when you begin to rely on something like alcohol to get you through social situations. I thought drinking would at least make me a bit more funny, or interesting.

Ellie Goulding

At 21, everyone's on Team Alcohol. It was the way I quieted my social anxiety. Drinking was like a quick phone-booth change into the charming extrovert the party demanded. I thought nothing of spending most evenings in a bar, because that's what my friends were doing. I thought nothing of mandating wine bottles for any difficult conversation—for any conversation at all—because that's what I saw in movies and television. Not taking a drink was easy. Just a matter of muscle movement, the simple refusal to put alcohol to my lips. The impossible part was everything else. How could I talk to people? Who would I be? When I cut out alcohol, my life got better. When I cut out alcohol, my spirit came back.

Sarah Hepola

Some people say, do you think you've missed out when you were younger not drinking and going out, but it never interested me much drinking, getting drunk. I'm not someone who needs to go out drinking to enjoy myself.

Harry Kane

I was not proud of myself getting drunk at 16 years old. The kids across the room who didn't drink, they had something I didn't have. Drinking just gave me this ability to be something else. … not be so rigid and uptight and worried and concerned. I could just kind of loosen up.

Chris Herren

I couldn't have relationships with people unless they drank as much as I drank. I didn't have deep relationships even with my family, because addiction gets in the way of all that. Most people did not know anything about my struggle with a brain disease. And so I found this great group of people that were struggling with the same things I struggled with. We got together. We spent a lot of time together. We focused on faith, service to others, truth, honesty, you know, all the things that are really important for being a human being of service and honesty. I still have those friends today. They're deeply embedded in my life and dear, dear, dear friends.

Kathryn Burgum

I was drunk 80% of the time. I loved it. In high school it was part of the culture. And in college, it was mandatory. And then when you get out of college people start to taper off. And I was surprised. I would look around and ask, 'Where are all my drunk buddies?' Everyone else had stopped drinking and I couldn't understand why.

David Letterman

My relationships were based on drinking. That's the only way I could have sex because I was scared of sex, and so I'd get blackout drunk. I don't think I'll ever drink again. I can dance now without it, I can have sex without it.

Nikki Glaser

I love London. It is in many ways my favorite city, but in certain circles, it can be very, very much about alcohol. You can easily have twelve drinks a day, and no one thinks you have a problem. Sometimes I'd say to my friends, 'I think I have a drinking problem' and they'd say, 'Oh, you don't have a drinking problem! Have another drink!'

Tom Ford

When my pals in high school were starting to drink, it always looked unappealing to me. I would be at a big party and see one of the popular girls or football players completely wasted and puking and acting a fool, and think to myself, 'There's nothing cool about that. I never wanted to be that out of control.

Kathy Griffin

I depended on alcohol to socialize with people. It was a bit of a crutch for me. And I lost a ton of friends who just didn't want to hang out with me because they didn't think it was fun anymore. So, that was an adjustment.

Amber Mac

Even though I would only drink once or twice a week, it was erratic. Sometimes I could have one and other times I could drink six, especially in social situations. I worked out it was social anxiety that really made me use alcohol to take the edge off those feelings. I thought I'd be boring or that I wouldn't be able to dance or have fun, but it's actually the opposite. I feel more confident because I'm fully there. The first time I went to an event unaided by alcohol was a challenge, but I showed myself that I didn't need alcohol to get through those situations.

Sarah Jane Clarke

I have never had a drink of alcohol in my life. I am a real outsider in my family. At a very young age I announced to everyone that I was never going to drink. It probably felt like a betrayal of my family and their entire legacy, but I have stuck to it.

Gillian Jacobs

I know many people would love for me to start drinking again. Everyone loved 'Party Kyle.' I think that was the hardest part of all of this. The resistance from others. But my mental and physical health became a lot more important to me than feeling like I had to be 'on' at a party or social setting. Even though I choose not to drink, I do entertain a lot and I want my guests to have nothing but the best.

Kyle Richards

I don't drink or party anymore. Clubs are no longer my scene. I can be around other people while they drink, but I don't want it. For a long, long time, the only thing that would help me put a smile on my face is if I was drinking. I was trying to drink myself into being someone else.

Mary J. Blige

I used to drink a lot in college. After a full day of school, I would get home and I would drink a bottle of wine and call it a day. I have done my fair share of drinking. I loved alcohol and it got to the point where even I started to, you know, cancel nights out that I felt like I wouldn't be able to control myself. It got harder for me to go out without having one drink to calm my nerves, which made me not want to go out at all, so I was just hibernating between jobs.

Bella Hadid

As soon as I turned 21, I was behind the bar. Bartending took the romanticism out of drinking. It ended after being on the other side of the bar. There is nothing sexy about a drunk girl. You really don't know how dumb you look. By the end of the time that I was bartending, it really disenchanted me with the whole idea of that whole scene.

Ronda Rousey

There's quite a lot of drinking involved in trail and ultra marathon running. We would run from pub to pub, me necking a half bottle of wine while the others had a beer. I'm proof alcoholics can hide in plain sight. I was so enslaved by drink I swigged wine during an ultramarathon. Alcohol is the only addictive substance that society will try and force on you against your will. It is the only addictive substance that people think you are odd, weird or broken if you don't take.

Allie Bailey

When I was younger, I was definitely going out too much and I was drinking too much. Alcohol is my drug of choice, and it was a gateway drug to other things for me. I'm clean and sober now, and I'm in a great place. I don't drink when I go to clubs. I'm in a different headspace. I don't want those things I wanted before. I feel better not drinking. It's more fun.

Lindsay Lohan

Not drinking hasn't been too tough on my social life and going out, as I don't have many friends. I mean that in a positive way. I have the friends I need and that's it.

Jessie J

I didn't want to get sober, I didn't like being around people who were. You laughed about the hangovers, and you laughed about, oh, I'm such a lush. And boy, it becomes unfunny, and it's unfunny when you're alone with yourself, and you have to come face to face with what it's doing to your soul. But sobriety gave me everything alcohol and drugs promised—belonging, self-respect, more laughter than you can even imagine, and profound companionship.

Anne Lamott

I outed myself as the poster girl for today's modern alcoholic, and she is female, well educated, professional, high functioning, and high bottom. So I got sober. I gave up drinking, and it was a new beginning. Switching off the impulse to drink turned out to be only one foot taking the step; fighting the culture around drinking was the other. We live in an alcogenic culture. The first question you're going to be asked is 'Red or white?'

Ann Dowsett Johnston

Nights out turned into endless calculations: How many glasses of wine has each person at this table had? What's the most of anyone? How much can I take, of what's left, without taking too much? With drinking, all my self-understanding hadn't granted me any release from compulsion. Removing alcohol was one of the best decisions I have made in my adult life.

Leslie Jamison

I don't have a problem saying what's on my mind without alcohol. Once a month, I would allow myself to go out to a party. I'd party once a month, but stayed away from drugs. That was never, never my thing. And so I drank, which you know eventually I realized wasn't my thing either. I don't drink and I care less if alcohol disappeared.

Andrew Huberman

I eventually stopped dating emotionally unavailable knobheads. I even learned how to dance in public sober. If I drink one, I want five. So now, I just don't have any. Once you see the world through sober eyes, it becomes clear that after one drink, most people are indeed looser, quicker to laugh, unclenched. However, at drink three that social alchemy begins to tarnish and rust. The looseness turns to sloppiness, the laughs become too loud, the jokes become muddled, quiet confidence turns to arrogance.

Catherine Gray

Although forgoing alcohol can be difficult, you'll never be sorry you made this decision. I had to quit drinking. I mean it was just not doing anything good for me and it ends by going to dark places in my family and the whole thing. Alcohol isn't the harmless habit many once believed. It's neurotoxic, addictive, and devastating for happiness and relationships. Substance abuse is the top predictor of marital breakdown and long-term unhappiness. If you want your later years to be your happiest years, guard your habits and stay vigilant about what you consume.

Arthur Brooks

The romance of wine clubs, scotch tastings, and 'a few beers while we watch the game' is dead for me. If you're asking yourself if your drinking is problematic, then, at the very least, drinking is probably not serving you. I see drinking culture as a great cover for pain.

Brené Brown

Many of my teammates were aware of my struggles with alcohol as my career approached its conclusion. That night getting arrested was one of the best things that has ever happened to me. Because if I don't get so publicly shamed and publicly humiliated, I don't think I wake up. I have not had a drink since that night I got arrested. So that night I was humiliated enough to wake up. It's really hard to talk about things when you're ashamed. And I'm not ashamed about what happened to me anymore. I'm proud of where I'm at.

Abby Wambach

I wasn't sold on not drinking yet because it's socially acceptable or whatever. The stigma around addiction keeps so many people suffering in silence. I want people to know there's no shame in asking for help. I felt better about my life at 11 months sober than I ever had playing in the NFL.

Darren Waller

Beer was the foundation of our alcoholic lifestyle. I played games when I was drunk. We were the boys of summer...an infamous rolling frat party. It became a lifestyle for me. So many celebrities go through what I went through with addiction and they end up dying because they never talk about their struggles. I have done that for years where I stuffed my feelings down and never really expressed how I feel.

Darryl Strawberry

Labeling myself as an alcoholic was one of the best things I had ever done, as opposed to just pretending like everything was okay. Everybody has issues that they have to deal with — some physical, some mental. This happens to be an issue of mine that I work on daily.

Steve Sarkisian

I've never been in a situation where I've been forced to drink. I myself don't want to drink and I don't want to try. It's just not a big deal for me. I myself don't want to drink and I don't want to try. It's not a big deal for me and I don't gravitate towards it.

Mohamed Salah

I owe it to myself and to my family to get myself right. When I was hiding all of this, it was isolating. I was worried nobody would understand. But now that it's out there, I don't have to live with that fear anymore. I didn't need to drink to have a good time. I am a good time. The people you are around, and your spirit is good enough. I never thought I could go five days without a drink. And yet, here I am.

CC Sabathia

I didn't drink to socialize. I drank to get drunk. I drank to escape. I wanted time to stop. I wanted the world to go away. In this new world of mine, I drank as often as I could. I would take four shots before even going out at night. At one point, I switched my drink of choice to vodka because the smell wasn't so easily detected

Sugar Ray Leonard

I don't drink anymore but back in the day, if I had two drinks after going to a party, then I'd take over the dance floor. Sachin asked me for a drink. I said I don't drink. He persisted. I said I don't drink. Eventually I said I will have four ice cubes. From then on it was pretty easy.

Virat Kohli

I was a binge drinker. When I drank, I drank to excess. It was what I did when I drank, the choices I made. I don't plan on drinking again. I can't think of one good thing alcohol ever did for me. Not one thing. I even listen to the guys talking about going out and I think, 'Am I supposed to be missing this?' Because I don't. Not once.

Brett Favre

I don't go out drinking and stuff like that. My friends say, 'Just have one drink, JD.' I say 'What's the point?' I'll go to a club and have a Red Bull. I dodged alcohol on nights out. I never drank a glass of spirits or wine until my wedding day. I don't drink, because I don't think I need to.

Jermain Defoe

From the moment I began drinking, I realized I was different from others. I couldn't simply enjoy one drink. I knew from Day 1 I couldn't just drink like everybody else. So, for me, I knew it was something that was always a crutch. I always knew I had a problem. I put my fiancée through hell and nobody knew… nobody believed her.

Maxx Crosby

I have never drunk alcohol & I never will. Back at school people would take the mick out of me for not drinking at parties and stuff, but that didn't bother me. As someone who doesn't drink, I love that no and low alcohol options like Heineken 0.0 allow me to enjoy a night out with friends, some great beer, and I still wake up feeling fresh – all while being the healthier choice too.

Gareth Bale

It was more important to have a drink than do anything. I was not treating myself or anyone around me with any respect. My best friends wouldn't let me on a session. It was all about me. That's all drugs and alcohol do, they cut off your emotions in the end. I was a drunk, but I'm not anymore. When I got sober, I had all this time and more energy.

Ringo Starr

I had a lot of issues at home, a lot of issues with my band. With alcohol, nothing was doing it for me and I decided I had to stop. . Alcohol makes you feel like you're having fun, but it's a lie.

Slash

When you stop drinking, you lose some things — but you gain a lot more. You fill your life with work and family and people you love. And honestly, that makes everything a lot easier.

John Mulaney

I have been abusive to myself and everyone around me for years. I have no excuses for my alcoholism or aggression, only rationalizations. Mel Gibson, Sean Penn, Josh Brolin — these guys got me to sobriety. They got around me and kept me alive. There were a bunch of guys that I looked up to that just started popping up. I had never, ever felt that kind of love — not like that.

Shia LaBeouf

It was 30 years of a disease that was taking its toll on everyone around me. It was getting to be too much. I got sober in L.A. and was anxious about coming home, but there are a lot of sober people out there. I found a community and a good network.

John Goodman

Personally, I've attended events and ceremonies where drinks were offered, but I chose not to take alcoholic drinks. Discipline in lifestyle means learning to say 'No.

Eliud Kipchoge

Just like a cancer patient needs chemotherapy to survive, an addict needs meetings and support to recover. It's a daily effort.

Doc Gooden

I don't need alcohol to be happy for one second. I've always been unbelievably comfortable with, like, 'Yo, this is how I roll'... not succumbing to any peer pressure in high school and college. Even though pretty girls were like, 'Come on, have a drink,' and even though my buddies were like, 'You're a puss, like, fucking drink,' it just didn't penetrate. It's now really wild for me to watch how many people don't want to drink anymore. It seems like the cool people don't want to drink. A lot more people are willing to say at like seven, ten, fifteen person gatherings, 'I don't drink.'

Gary Vaynerchuk

I think it's weird that people think it's weird I don't drink alcohol. Poisoning yourself intentionally is a weird flex IMHO, but I support your right to do so.

Casey Neistat

Whether in high school or college, whenever I found myself in a situation in which everybody was drinking, I always thought of my dad. Because someone that I respected so highly had chosen to not drink, I could make the same choice with confidence. I didn't mind guys drinking, but what I do mind is our society's inability to see alcohol for what it truly is: a drug.

Tony Dungy

I don't drink and hang out anymore. If I ever felt like going out and dancing, I could do it. I could sit around everybody while they're drinking, but I just don't want to.

Mary J Blige

I was a mess. I was drinking vodka out of the bottle, no ice, no glass, nothing, and I couldn't stop. Alcoholism is a lonely disease. You're scared to death of being alone, but you're also scared to let anybody really get to know you. I had burned a lot of bridges. I had done crazy things. I didn't really have any friends—nobody in the music business could really count on me to do anything. I just kind of isolated and sat at home, and I had my own little universe that I was the head of. The only thing that mattered was not running out of vodka and cocaine. And that was a lot of work. I thought I was going to drown in a bathtub in some hotel alone somewhere like all my buddies had.

Joe Walsh

I'm approaching my third year of sobriety, and I've just got back from a meeting actually. If I don't go, then I end up in Shit Street. I've reached a really weird place with it. I'm not really happy being sober, but I don't want to get drunk. Someone told me that at three years sober they felt exactly the same.

Ozzy Osbourne

I thought I would never be funny again. I thought I would lose my creativity. I thought sober people were like a cult who sold books at the airport. I don't think there were any bands that even knew what sober was. We believed that the road to wisdom was through excess. But getting clean was the hardest — and best — thing I've ever done. I keep myself surrounded by the people that are sober, and I rely on them for things in my life.

Steven Tyler

I thought there was something otherworldly about the whole culture of drinking, that being drunk made me a member of some strange, mysterious club. I was a practicing alcoholic.

Eric Clapton

I don't drink. I don't want to stand around and listen to drunk people tell me a story.

RuPaul

I was barely 21, and I was a full-blown alcoholic. I was drinking all the time. Getting sober was not easy for me. The first six months of getting sober consisted of nothing but accumulative isolation. My phone stopped ringing the minute word got out that I had put the bottle down — and that was pretty painful.

Kat Von D

I drank with people like Jimi Hendrix and Jim Morrison. You were just drinking beer with the boys. I was the most functional alcoholic on the planet. You never knew I was drunk. But I was drinking more and more. I loved my life, but I hated my life. I became an alcoholic. Didn't realize I was going to become an alcoholic. There's nothing cool about being a drunk. I am now the classic example of a rock star who doesn't drink, doesn't smoke, and doesn't do drugs.

Alice Cooper

Seven months sober. That's a lot of sober flights. A lot of sober conversations. I don't find interest in partying anymore... maybe I'm changing and that's deeper than alcohol.

Ari Lennox

I admit I struggled with alcohol and it weighed heavily on me. When you get drunk, you're not how you usually are. The more and more I see it on other people, the more and more it makes me happy about the decision.

Allen Iverson

After 15 or 20 years of carousing the way I caroused and drinking the way I drank, the sober world is a pretty scary world. To come home and not to have the buffer support of a few drinks just to calm the nerves, it was a really amazing thing. And I remember being more nervous, and being more uncomfortable because I didn't have any booze. I don't have sober friends, I really don't.

Colin Farrell

A decade ago I wasn't booking many jobs so I would party all the time, drink, smoke and hang out with people who were a bad influence. I got clean and sober and learned I was an alcoholic and that there was a whole world out there that lived sober. I met some amazing people in recovery who helped me find myself without alcohol.

Elsa Hosk

In terms of navigating being in the public eye, I think sobriety is the best thing I ever did. But the first year that I stopped, I felt like I'd really lost a big part of who I was. Sobriety was really lonely at the beginning. Partying was, I felt, a defining feature of my personality. Once I drank, the alcohol would just tell me what to do, or who I was hanging out with, or whatever, and I had no real independence with it. It sort of ruled my whole life.

Florence Welch

At public dinners I sometimes drink a glass of champagne or perhaps two. On the average, I may drink one glass of champagne a month. It is of incalculable consequence to the man himself that he should be sober and temperate. I have never drunk whiskey or brandy except when the doctor prescribed it I have never been drunk or in the slightest degree under the influence of liquor.

Theodore Roosevelt

At one point, I could never have conceived of going out and not drinking, but as time goes on, you lose the urge and the insecurity that often makes people drink in the first place.

Gerard Butler

I was often by myself, drinking alone, waking up in the morning and having a vodka tonic in the shower. I was working as a lawyer, and trying to sneak drinks throughout the day. It was exhausting. It was sad and lonely. I had burned bridges with friends. I was unreliable. My parents didn't want anything to do with me. And ultimately I had a marriage that ended on the honeymoon. I created a lot of chaos and wreckage, and destroyed a lot of relationships. If my story stands for anything, it is that the human body, mind, and spirit are far more resilient than you can possibly imagine. Recovery is possible.

Rich Roll

I quit drinking when I was 27, had a brief attempt to drink socially again around 50, saw the same stupidity in myself, and dropped it completely. If I go out and watch people drink now, it just makes everyone look stupid and foggy minded. Alcohol rarely brings out the best in people; it often pushes them into versions of themselves they later regret.

Jordan Peterson

I stopped drinking alcohol many years ago and I have more fun than ever. I don't need a drug to be courageous or to dance You're not partying; you're killing yourself. You think alcohol is your friend, but it's the enemy. It's taking everything from you.

Jocko Willink

The biggest reason I don't consume alcohol is because if I have a glass of wine, I don't want to be responsible for a kid looking up to me and saying, 'Hey, Tebow's doing' it — I am going to do it.' And then he makes a bad decision. Because, like it or not, it is serious.

Tim Tebow

As much as I would love to be a person that goes to parties and has a couple of drinks and has a nice time, that doesn't work for me. I do that very unsuccessfully. I'd just rather sit at home and read, or go out to dinner with someone, or talk to someone I love, or talk to somebody that makes me laugh. I'm more comfortable now, knowing I'm someone who enjoys just hanging out with my friends . . . I used to wonder, 'Am I boring for not wanting to go out and get drunk all the time?

Daniel Radcliffe

I became sober at the age of 29, and now I've maintained that for 19 years. I've been incredibly fortunate. I wouldn't have been able to have access to myself or other people, or even been able to take in other people, if I hadn't changed my life. I never would have been able to have the relationships that I do. I never would have been able to take care of my father the way I did when he was sick. So many things.

Bradley Cooper

I think the first month I was like, I'm going to give it a month, just see if I feel any better, and if my interactions with those that are closest to me improve. And they did. And I'm like, all right, I'm going to go another month. And then it got traction. I had momentum.

Charlie Sheen

I feel like I was carrying this version of myself that I had been since I was 20, 21... and it was no longer serving who I was to become. As a musician you go to a lot of festivals and club appearances and shows, and where there's music there's usually alcohol and drugs. It's always around. But I wasn't liking the person that was reflecting back at me, and I was like, 'OK, I think it's time to, like, sober up,' and I need to just get away from people and figure out who am I right now.

Doechii

I didn't hit a rock bottom. I just got tired of digging...Tired of digging myself out of messes. I just felt like, "This isn't the full me. I was great at work, but then I wasn't fully present when I finally go home, because when I go home, I gotta have a couple drinks.

Lane Kiffin

I've been sober for five and a half years now and it gets a lot easier. I had to learn the hard way that I can't do parties anymore.

Demi Lovato

Everything in moderation is a dance with the devil. I saw people high or tipsy and it just seemed so unnecessary and unauthentic... it seemed like manufactured fabricated fun. I've found it's far better and more productive to just say no, no thank you.

Steve Harvey

5. Quotes on the Success Side

Productivity, Capacity, Full Potential, Aspirations

I can trace my success from that moment I stopped drinking. Because I don't drink, I'm killing it. My life changed. I saw all the comics that got the most work done weren't drinking; the most successful ones didn't drink. It wasn't a fix-all for me, but I think it was the greatest decision I ever made for me.

Nikki Glaser

My success directly correlates to me getting straight and me getting in touch with who I am and understanding what my talents were and how to tap into them in a positive way. So I was doing things the right way, it was just that one thing that was in the way – my addiction. And once that was out of the way, it was – boom! The door blew wide open.

Samuel L. Jackson

I looked out the window and went, "OK, John, what percentage of your potential would you like to have?" Because if you say you'd like 60, and you'd like to spend the other 40 having fun, that's fine. But what percentage of what is available to you would you like to make happen? There's no wrong answer. What is it? I went, "100."

John Mayer

I didn't just want to be sober; I wanted to be better. I sought help, embraced sobriety and the rest is aquatic history. Within six months of breaking my addiction, at age 31, I was breaking masters world records. Within a year I was swimming personal lifetime bests. I have been sober for 23 years now since my return to swimming. Swimming was my sanctuary, but sobriety was my salvation.

Karlyn Pipes

Getting sober just exploded my life. Now I have a much clearer sense of myself and what I can and can't do. I am more successful than I have ever been. I feel very positive where I never did before, and I think that's all a direct result of getting sober.

Jamie Lee Curtis

I always wanted to see how far I could go in the sport. I didn't want to do anything to jeopardize that. I made some mistakes when I was 16 or 17 in Barcelona, but now I don't go out, I don't drink, I don't smoke and none of the top players do.

Andy Murray

I realized I wasn't going to live up to my potential, and that scared the hell out of me. I thought, 'Wow, I'm actually going to ruin my life.' The one thing that I've learned in life is the best thing I can do is embrace who I am and then do that to the fullest extent, and then whatever happens, happens. The more steps I do to not do that, the farther I am away from fulfilling any potential I would have.

Bradley Cooper

I wanted to be more successful. The top-performing people I've ever been around, they are very against alcohol, against substances. And they'll tell you they perform better. They think clearly. They have better memory, better recall, more energy, and are more precise.

Charlie Kirk

So what do you get when you combine tons of extra free time, more clarity and focus, and a stronger commitment to building things in your life that are going to last long term? You get the biggest fucking productivity boost imaginable. Look, I've tried all the hacks. I've done the morning routines. I did the sauna and coal plunge shit. I tried every productivity system under the sun. No system, no book, no hack can beat a highly functioning metabolism, a great night of sleep, and a genuine excitement to work on something over the long term.

Mark Manson.

Being sober means that I operate better and I function better; I believe I am meant to be that way. Choosing not to drink has been one of the biggest acts of self-respect in my life. The longer I stayed sober, the more I realized how small alcohol had been making my world.

Rumer Willis

I knew I wasn't at my full potential, and that's what was starting to get to me. I felt 'enslaved' by my addiction, and I was 'living a very, very small life.' I had to make a decision to go and make the changes necessary to get sober. It's something I needed because I'm alcoholically wired. I wish I'd gotten sober many years earlier than I did, but it is what it is.

Keith Urban

Stopping drinking is probably the most powerful personal development strategy which I've ever found. I just hit 1,000 days without drinking alcohol. I've built three businesses, bought five houses, traveled to fifteen countries, and learned a ton of lessons about myself and life in general since I went sober.

Chris Williamson

I don't have time to waste. If you're toasted you need a day to recover. You get a hangover. So that's two days out of your life. Let's say there are 365 days in a year, so in 10 years that's 3650, so how many days do you want to waste?

Denzel Washington

I don't want to lose time—you know, if you have a night out, you lose the days following. I'll suffer for several days — sometimes it'll be like three or four days. I've always been looking for how do you get that extra 1%. As an athlete, that's what you are always doing.

Lewis Hamilton

I don't drink alcohol. It's poison for your body. If you want to be the best, you have to sacrifice. My body is my temple. My career is my life. I play clean. I live clean. I do this not just for me but for my kids, my mom and my family.

Cristiano Ronaldo

What I don't have to deal with is any of the baggage. No hangovers. Fewer embarrassing losses of self-control. No awkward apologies. No large bar tabs (unless I'm buying, which happens often enough). No DUIs, nor a worry about how I might get home somewhere. All of these little bonuses added up. Looking back, I see they were instrumental in succeeding at an early age by the way—of getting an edge on the competition. While my peers had a nightly habit to support or a crutch they depended on, I didn't.

Ryan Holiday

When I began to write seriously, I had to quit drinking, because I simply could not think clearly enough while hungover. By my mid-twenties I realized it was either the serious writing or the drinking, and I chose to let the drinking go.

Jordan Peterson

It isn't "sobriety made me perfect." It's "sobriety made my life possible." I have to contribute sobriety a hundred percent to my success right now. A lot of people say, 'Oh my God, you're so articulate,' or, 'You can really express yourself.' And I learned that all through recovery, just being in the rooms, sharing my experience, strength and hope. I was afraid I wouldn't be creative if I was sober. It seemed all the cool and creative people were drinking. It's not true.

Kevin Kreider

I started writing right when I got sober after being lost to food and alcohol addiction for a very long time. I found the magic of recovery.

Glennon Doyle

I made a change at age 25 that transformed my life forever. I quit doing weekends. I quit drinking. I quit smoking. I quit trying to impress people. I quit making excuses. Five years… that's what it took from getting out of rehab to making my first million.

Grant Cardone

I was tired of pretending that alcohol was making life easier when really it was holding me back. I tried to moderate my drinking for six years, and it was only when I really tried to properly stop that I realized how hard it was. Quitting wasn't about giving something up—it was about coming back to who I really am. Not relying on drinking made me rely on the qualities and skills I actually have.

Jay Shetty

Getting sober really kind of turned my brain back on. An unexpected side effect of getting sober was I'm motivated: I feel like I've lost some time and I want to make up for that. My disease cost me a big chunk of my life and career. I wasted a lot of time. I romanticized the idea of alcohol. I'm not saying it didn't provide great moments of great escape and relief and easing of pain, but it wound up creating chaos and destroying things — destroying creativity in my case. After getting sober, there was an awkward adjustment of learning how to live without drugs or alcohol. Once I got on stable ground and started to understand how my brain worked without all that... I can do more because I can remember what I did. I can think deeper about things.

Trent Reznor

Alcohol absolutely works for a while, but suddenly it starts influencing your greatness. When I got sober I started writing even better. All the magic that you thought worked when you were high comes out when you get sober. You realize it was always there, and your fear goes away. We all got sober, I guess, over '88, '89, and those albums were all off the charts. Finally had a No. 1 single.

Steven Tyler

Once I stopped drinking I found this clarity, which can be painful for a while but my life has just fallen into place. I built a business, made a movie, had a child, I'm making another movie.

Tom Ford

I am running circles around every younger version of myself. it's all because of sobriety. It's truly nuts that I'm celebrating a full sixteen years of sobriety today.

Steve O.

Sobriety gave me more time to work, and more focus. And, you know, it made my career happen. It gave me everything, really, that I have now. If I hadn't have been in a car accident, I probably could have maintained for quite a few years. And I would probably have been a struggling songwriter and touring musician, and probably would have thought that my music was just going over everybody's head. Or I was born too late: all these excuses that people give when your work is not quite strong enough or when they don't work hard enough or aren't able to focus. And I would have just kept on drinking and kept on ruining relationships. I don't think I would have my wife and my daughter, and I certainly wouldn't have a big pile of Grammys and all that kind of shit.

Jason Isbell

I think you get more out of yourself if you don't drink. Everyone knows I don't drink alcohol. All along I've tried not to get in that habit of drinking because you don't need it if you want to keep performing at the highest level for a long time. That's probably why I'm still playing to be honest. When I finish playing one day I can say to myself 'you know I did everything right'.

Jermain Defoe

I do believe that I would never have been able to direct a major studio movie if I hadn't stopped. There are things that I'm doing in my life now that I don't think that I would've been able to sustain. It [alcohol] affects everything, and that's part of the reason why I stopped, because even if you're going out a couple of times a week and you're drinking, it was starting to affect me throughout the week

Sanaa Lathan

I got sober when I was 20. It's been 10 years of no drinking. Being sober for me didn't mean that my life came to an end. It was the beginning of a real, beautiful, big, happy successful life. It's ok not to drink or do drugs. It's the best decision I ever made. Sobriety taught me about showing up and being accountable.

Elsa Hosk

You see, even though back when I was drinking I thought nothing bad ever happened to me, something did. Time passed. A lot of time passed. So actually, something bad, very bad, did happen to me. I wasted my life. And now, what little I have left, I want. And If I was going to be completely sober for the rest of my life… then the life I lived needed to be a life from which I did not seek escape. I've certainly accomplished a lot, and I accomplished everything because I don't drink. That's the only variable. Nothing else in my life changed except I stopped drinking.

Augusten Burroughs

I tried drinking at 26 for the first time. Alcohol was awesome, and I loved it. I just don't let myself do it because there are just too many downsides. So I *get* how people get in trouble. So for me it was easy to be like, "Yeah, this is fun," but I can weigh it against the disadvantages. And there are way too many.

Tom Bilyeu

When I used to drink, I lived mostly in my head. I would imagine all the things I wanted to do and make elaborate plans, but never actually managed to make or do anything concrete in the real world. Now when I have an idea, I'm able to make it happen. There's something to show for the time that is passing. I'm living in my real life, not just imagining it. Strangely, life now is no less intense than it was when I was partying hard in my early 20s, it's just more authentic, and more productive.

Hayley Gibson

Sober is a superpower. Because when you can't reach for alcohol to give you courage, you have to reach inside yourself instead. There will come a point, after about 100 days, when you are FREE. And then your life will start to transform in so many ways.

Clare Pooley

I quit drinking in my twenties because I knew I was never going to reach my potential with that in my life. I got into the acting program, it was very challenging, I was hungover and I wasn't doing so well in my classes. I realized it was not going to end well. I thought, 'Do you know what? It's going to be one or the other. I can't really have both. Acting is the only thing that made me want to ever get sober. Because my love for acting was so big when I was very young, I had something that was more important to me than just drinking. It was enough of a problem for me to go, 'This is something that could get in the way of what I want to do in life.' I've been sober since 22 — and I got sober so I could act.

Kristin Davis

Sobriety gives you an unbelievable edge in life. Sobriety will enable you to become the man you always wanted to be. You will find your life's purpose from your struggles.

Chris Herren

I'll actually enjoy my life by going to sleep, rather than going to a club. 80 per cent of athletes drink alcohol, so a lot needs to be done. ' I try to say no to anything which is not beneficial. Discipline in lifestyle means learning to say 'No. What made me stay at the top for a long time is self-discipline.

Eliud Kipchoge

I don't drink or smoke. I'm trying to win. You don't have to be a 'problem drinker' for alcohol to hurt you. It's an addictive depressant, even in moderation. Alcohol has destroyed more lives than I can count...that's why I don't think people should drink. You're only squandering your whole future and your potential when you let alcohol run your life.

Jocko Willink

June second, 1977. If you want the truth, I'm prouder of that, that I've quit drinking, than I am of anything in my life. I don't see anything coming out of my drinking experiences except waste and pain and misery. Booze takes a lot of time and effort.

Raymond Carver

There are fighters in America who can drink on Friday and Saturday. After an event I saw it myself in the hotel -- 80 percent of them are already drunk. Not the champs, but middle-of-the-pack guys, guys like one win, two losses. I don't drink. I never drink. You want a better life? Start with better habits.

Khabib Nurmagomedov

I'd always thought that if I could get sober and stay sober, I would be able to have a career making music. It was the one thing that was holding me back. When I'm sober, I'm prolific and productive. When I get sober something magical happens again. If I want to make music then I have to be sober. Without treatment, I wouldn't have a music career.

Macklemore

I had everything in my life I could have ever wanted. I had money. I had fame and, for some reason, when I got there and I got everything that I wanted, I think that was truly the most empty I had ever felt inside. I was self-medicating with alcohol. That's what I thought would make me happy. Alcohol was detrimental to where I was trying to go in my life. I really didn't see that until it was too late. What did that get me? Where did that get me except out of the NFL? Where did that get me? Disgraced?

Johnny Manziel

It wasn't until boxing when I physically had to fight someone else that I had to be sober and I had to focus that I felt better. It was like this giant wake up call. Boxing saved me from a drinking problem. It's made my life exponentially better — just more sharp, more focused, clearer thinking, and then for sure on the athletic side with what it does to your body.

Jake Paul

I had to make a clear decision. I just wanted more, and I deserved more, and I could achieve more. I want to be sober for the rest of my life — that's something I work at every day.

Gregory Gourdet

While I certainly don't ever push the sober life on others, I'm more than happy to discuss my journey and why I owe much of my success to this lifestyle. Since quitting drinking, I have been grateful to wake up with a clear mind. I hated the feeling of being hungover and not having clarity.

Amber Mac

I wasn't a 'rock bottom' alcoholic, but I was definitely a gray-area drinker. Alcohol was just always there. Since I stopped drinking, my creative channels have opened up in a way I didn't expect. I'm much more focused on my brand. My energy levels are much higher, my sleep is better, and I feel like I have more time in the day.

Sarah Jane Clarke

Stopping drinking was the first step but it was only the beginning. What came next was looking at all the other toxic parts of my life. Healing. Facing the things I had avoided for so long. Slowly stepping into my power. Positives for me really are the time that I've got back, the time that I'm not spent hungover.

Millie Mackintosh

I just really felt like alcohol wasn't serving me. I didn't have a problem with alcohol, per se... but it really was a choice for health and beauty. I wanted to look and feel my best. All I know is I have never felt better physically or been more clear mentally. I'm exercising and not drinking, because guess what, even if I have two glasses of wine, the next day I feel down and depressed. I can't afford to be depressed right now. I feel fantastic, so I don't see the point right now.

Kyle Richards

I was touring with Bruno Mars, and I definitely was drinking too much. I was a bit out of control. I wasn't happy. I thought drinking would at least make me a bit more funny, or interesting. I had to be a fake person to deal with the surreal situation I was in. I assumed I couldn't be good enough, smart, funny, or crazy enough to be with certain people without it. It's scary when you begin to rely on something like alcohol to get you through social situations. I was – you know, I can see it in my performances that I wasn't good. I would drink before going on stage, I thought it would calm my nerves, but it actually made things so much worse. I can't have a big night out before a show anymore. I'm protective of my voice and my body now.

Ellie Goulding

I like my life to be pure and clean and organized, and I like to have had eight hours' sleep a night. I honestly don't think I'd be as successful if I was a party animal. Because I don't think my personality would be as focused and open as it is.

Jessie J

It really had control over me. I just felt like I was no longer in control of my own destiny. I wasn't liking the person that was reflecting back at me, and I was like, 'Okay, it's time to stop and sober up.' My life has never been as fulfilling as it is now. Everything is going well, and I believe that wouldn't be the case if I weren't sober.

Lily Allen

Alcohol made my life smaller. It made my world smaller. It made me smaller. Calling myself sober, and not ingesting ethanol on the regular, led to greater clarity, and also a mad desire to break through all the limitations I had accepted for my life.

Holly Whitaker

Alcohol is a deceptive drug. It creates the illusion of pleasure and relaxation while causing the very anxiety and discomfort it purports to relieve. When I was drinking, I mean, I really felt like I couldn't cope with my life. I felt like it was all too hard. And anything extra at all I just couldn't cope with when I was drinking.

William Porter

Beneath my own witty, professional facade were oceans of fear, whole rivers of self-doubt. When I drank, the part that felt dangerous and needy grew bright and strong and real. But in some deep and important personal respects you stop growing when you start drinking alcoholically. The drink stunts you. For a long time, when it's working, the drink feels like a path to a kind of self-enlightenment, something that turns us into the person we wish to be, or the person we think we are. In some ways the dynamic is simple: alcohol makes everything better, until it makes everything worse. You don't realize how badly you're in trouble until you try to get out of it.

Caroline Knapp

People who quit drinking become terrified they will lose their power. They believe booze makes them the people they want to be. A better mother. A better lover. A better friend. Alcohol is one hell of a pitchman, and perhaps his greatest lie is convincing us we need him, even as he tears us apart. I needed to build a new tolerance. In need to say Yes to discomfort, yes to frustration, yes to failure, because it meant I was getting stronger. I had to refuse to be the person who only played games she could win. That is true strength.

Sarah Hepola

I quit drinking alcohol in my 30s, and I did a lot of things differently than I hadn't done before, because I wanted to not have the future that I saw coming. If you drink at night, and if you want to be productive the next morning, this morning starts last night, and it starts by going to bed at a reasonable time sober. Zero alcohol is better for individuals than any alcohol. For those not prone to alcohol use disorder and of age, probably two drinks per week should be the upper ceiling.

Arthur Brooks

My life was way worse because of alcohol. I knew that I was struggling with my drinking. I knew that I needed to quit. Those that know me, know that I have always demanded excellence from myself. I've been sober for almost nine, for nine years now and everything really powerfully good in my life has happened in my sobriety.

Abby Wambach

Now eight years sober, the mere fact that I'm standing on the sideline as a College Football Playoff head coach could serve as inspiration to anyone going through what I experienced. I came out of it all knowing there was a better version of Steve Sarkisian inside of me.

Steve Sarkisian

Nutrition is so important; it's part of the game. It has helped with my recovery, allowed me to sleep better, and helped my body adapt quickly. I myself don't want to drink and I don't want to try. It's not a big deal for me and I don't gravitate towards it.

Mohamed Salah

Training is vital, but living a calm life is just as important so you can be at your best physically and mentally; I spend my free time with family and friends to stay relaxed and positive.

Cristiano Ronaldo

I came to play football, not to drink alcohol. I don't drink, I don't smoke, I don't have tattoos. I don't want to impress anyone, I just want to show the best of myself on the pitch. I won't touch alcohol, religion is very important to me.

Sadio Mané

My training was horrible, I ate so bad, I was up until late, I was having a drink or two regularly. It was a horrible mindset. When I started my fitness turnaround, it was more of a lifestyle thing initially. In the middle of 2012, just after the IPL, I realized I need to make changes in my physical condition and fitness levels. That was a lifestyle choice. Now there is no room for late night binges, spontaneous cheat days or emotional eating. What you eat affects your temperament, focus, confidence, and sleep.

Virat Kohli

During the season I don't drink. And to be honest it doesn't really interest me. It never interested me much drinking, getting drunk. I can't remember the last time I went to a club.

Harry Kane

Alcohol and drugs are like a solvent. When I put it in my body, things start to disappear. Wives, kids, jobs, homes, cars, everything disappears. People always ask me, you know, what's your greatest accomplishment in life? And I say, my sobriety. Without my sobriety, I got nothing. Today I celebrate 20 years of sobriety. What a journey it has been.

Theo Fleury

My journey in sobriety is my badge of honor, not my shameful story. It got to a point after my rookie year my life became unmanageable. Alcohol, partying and all that shit became too much of a distraction in my life. It became just overwhelming. and I was close to losing everything – my career, my health, my relationships. I had to go to rehab in the offseason, and I needed help. It was the best thing I ever did. I'm a completely different person.

Maxx Crosby

In terms of navigating being in the public eye, I think sobriety is the best thing I ever did. I really bought into the myth that the chaos was all part of your creativity. However, after getting sober, I found it to be absolutely the opposite. When I realized I could perform without the booze it was a revelation. The more peaceful I am, the more I can give to the work.

Florence Welch

All that energy I was putting towards self-destruction I just put towards music. Alcohol was the one thing that was destroying my life. It was all about the next drink, the next fix. It was all just chaos and destruction.

Slash

Sobriety comes before anything else in my life. If I use drugs or alcohol, I will lose my family, my band, my house, my financial security. Sobriety has given me all of those things and more. Sobriety allows me to look at life and go, 'I want to be a good man. I want to be a good friend. I want to be a good husband. I want to be a good father and I want to be a good musician.'

Nikki Sixx

All the pitfalls that people read about, I just found myself slipping into all of them. Mostly, like, substance abuse. I've worked my whole life to get to where I am, and you can't lose all of it over something that you do in your spare time. I can't work under the influence. I can't write songs under the influence. I can't perform under the influence.

Ed Sheeran

I drank right through until I was 34. And I had the show at NBC and I just said to myself, 'You're a fool, you're a dumb fool. You can't do this. You know, they just don't give these shows to everybody. You have one. And you drink yourself into trouble, you're done, pal!' And I just quit. Never took another drink. I realized that drinking every night was an impediment, it could be an encumbrance, and I would never forgive myself if I drank away this opportunity.

David Letterman

It was an innate knowing, this idea that I was saying no to something bigger by choosing to drink and spend my time that way, and it grew as time went on. It was the less urgent but more convincing argument to me. Sobriety is not just about not drinking. It's about peeling back the layers and getting to the core of who you are.

Laura McKowen

I've got to look at my failures in the face for a while. I need to take ownership of my shit and clean up my side of the street a bit before I can go out there and work again. I'm trying to stay creative and learn from my mistakes. The truth is, in my desperation, I lost the plot.

Shia LaBeouf

If I'm perfectly honest, without my career and without that creative outlet, I don't know if I would've made it. I think that show and my love of what I do was my North Star truly, it really gave me purpose, and still gives me purpose. But I was constantly in this cycle of extreme depression and anxiety while having to show up to work and be on. And that 'being on' fueled even more drinking. I was caught in this cycle that I couldn't get out of.

Lucy Hale

I've made my life more stressful by drinking and using drugs. I was even drinking at work. My cheeks would turn bright red and my speech would get slurred. It's a miracle anyone would hire me. I looked like a walking heart attack. I know I'm a slow learner, but, by God, I've learned. I always think of the downtimes, how it made me feel, how I fouled up everything I ever did in my life.

John Goodman

I don't drink or smoke. I'm trying to win. You don't have to be a 'problem drinker' for alcohol to hurt you. It's an addictive depressant, even in moderation. You're only squandering your whole future and your potential when you let alcohol run your life. Alcohol has destroyed more lives than I can count.

Jocko Willink

Alcohol doesn't fit into my life. It just is so incredibly… it's so unproductive. It's like the opposite of everything I love, which is like accomplishments and doing things and self-improvement. If you care about getting things done, drinking is the enemy.

Casey Neistat

I stopped immediately when I realized I could lose my voice or I could lose my career over this. I chose to learn how to drink socially and it didn't work. The test comes when you have to decide whether you're drinking to be social or drinking to get drunk.

Mary J Blige

It was starting to extract a greater toll, energetically. I could tell it was preventing me from reaching as far as I could, creatively and physically. All I know is, I could feel its presence in an ominous, daunting way that was preventing me from being my higher self.

Ben Harper

I had forgotten I was a musician. I forgot I play guitar—just didn't do that anymore. I just kind of isolated and sat at home, We were on top of the world with the Eagles, and we were wild and crazy. That was okay back then, in the late '70s. And in 1980, we just ran out of steam. After about 15 years, Don Henley and Glenn Frey came to me and said: "We have been thinking of starting the Eagles back up again, and we can't do it without you, and we can't do it unless you're sober." I was just about homeless. If I got sober, the Eagles would be back together. And I said to myself, "Man, if I'm going to do this, this is my chance." I said, 'Well, I can get sober for that.' That's a darn good reason. And it was a godsend. I didn't get sober for me at first. I got sober so I could show up and be in the Eagles again. And then I stayed sober for me. People tell me I play better now sober than I did before.

Joe Walsh

My life had become a catastrophe. I had no idea how to turn it around. My band had broken up. I had almost lost my family. My whole life had devolved into a disaster. I believe that the police officer who stopped me at three a.m. that morning saved my life. The minute I got arrested, I was relieved. I knew it was over. I've been sober since January 5, 2007. I'm happy to be sober. Happy to be alive. My children are happy. In August, my wife and I will celebrate our fifteenth wedding anniversary. My band is back together with a sold-out tour.

Trey Anastasio

I was hanging out with people a lot older than me, and I was looking at their lives, and so at 19 I was like, "I don't want to be like you when I'm 30. I don't want to be like any of you. I'm super-ambitious, I want to be working, and I want to do something meaningful with my life. So I got sober at 19. I gained a lot of clarity into what I was capable of accomplishing when my head was sober and focused on the greater good. Work became easy, and everything that was on my dream list since I'm a kid, I've done.

Soko

I thought that if I stopped drinking and I stopped using drugs, I would not be able to play. It was very frightening, the idea of getting sober. Once I managed to get sober, I realized drugs and alcohol were a shortcut to inspiration – a detriment. If I'd known that earlier, it might have brought me to recovery sooner. If I have any regret, it's that musically I lost something there.

Eric Clapton

It's a real, real gift, this sobriety. You honor that gift by shining, by showing up as the best version of yourself.

RuPaul

By the time I was 34, I was really entrenched in a lot of trouble. But there were years that I was sober during that time. Season 9 was the year that I was sober the whole way through. And guess which season I got nominated for best actor? I was like, 'That should tell me something. The thing is, if I don't have sobriety, I don't have anything.

Everything starts with sobriety. Because if you don't have sobriety, you're going to lose everything that you put in front of it.

Matthew Perry

I didn't think I had a problem because I wasn't drinking every day. But when I would drink an alcoholic drink, I wanted another one, and another one, and another one, and another one. And it was holding me back from my full potential. I needed to better my life.

Blac Chyna

My live shows are a million times better now. If you drink, you can't even remember if it's a good show or not — and that's probably for the best, because it would have been rubbish because I'd have been drunk and not making any sense.

Calvin Harris

Everybody else can do what they want, but that stuff isn't for me. I just don't want to drink. You can't get anything done hanging out all day long.

Pharrell Williams

The first and most seductive peril, and the destroyer of most young men, is the drinking of liquor. You are more likely to fail in your career from acquiring the habit of drinking liquor than from... other temptations.

Andrew Carnegie

I was somebody who started out with a lot of promise. I was the kid who graduated at the top of my class in high school. I got into every college I applied to—Harvard, Princeton. I went on to Stanford, where I was a member of the legendary Stanford swimming program. I was a world-class swimmer. I vividly remember the feeling of being drunk for the very first time. It was as if I was being encased in a warm blanket, and everything that was anxiety-provoking in my life seemed to vanish. It was all fun and games, and I was having a great time in college partying. But it was a slow progression that started to monopolize my interest, meanwhile eroding other aspirations I had in my life. And so it became paramount, and just monopolized everything that I was doing. Alcohol stole my life. My focus narrowed to only that which was right in front of me. In other words, Where is my next good time?

Rich Roll

Just because I'm now the legal drinking age, doesn't mean I'm going to start throwing 'em back. I don't plan to start drinking. My life is too stressful to need help with relaxing by having a cocktail. This industry is way too nuts for me to not be in control of myself and my decisions, so I just don't want to introduce drinking! Plus, I don't want drinking to become a vice. Why try something if you don't need it?!

Zendaya

One of the biggest reasons for me to stop drinking was to preserve and protect my art. During my drinking years, I was acutely aware that I could be operating at a much more proficient level if I could just eliminate these distractions. There're so many more beautiful things to be inspired by in the world.

Kat Von D

There is no way anyone can perform at their best if they're dulling their brain with alcohol or drugs. I've always felt that if you want to win in anything that really matters, you need every bit of clarity and sharpness you can get, so I stay away from anything that interferes with that.

Larry Ellison

I doubt I'd be standing here if I hadn't quit drinking whiskey, and beer and wine and all that. Quitting drinking was one of the toughest decisions I have ever made. Without it, none of the others that follow would have been possible. I had too much to drink one night. The next day I decided to quit and I haven't had a drink since.

George W. Bush

The idea that the creative endeavor and mind-altering substances are entwined is one of the great pop-intellectual myths of our time. ... Substance abusing writers are just substance abusers — common garden variety drunks and druggies.

Stephen King

It's a great advantage not to drink among hard drinking people.

F. Scott Fitzgerald

Twelve years ago today, I got sober. I stopped killing myself with alcohol. I began to think: Wait a minute — if I can stop doing this, what are the possibilities? A significant benefit of maintaining sobriety is the freedom from occupying your mind with thoughts about alcohol consumption.

Dax Shepard

Alcohol and the craft of acting is not a smart combination. Nobody gives you a shoulder to cry on because you seem to have so much — like money and fame. Alcohol breeds self-pity and I've resorted to it on and off throughout my life. But I kicked it by making other things more important.

Patrick Swayze

Emerging from treatment felt akin to being reborn. I was completely stripped down and incredibly exposed. It was like embarking on a new life with an entirely different set of guidelines. I experienced anxiety about my ability to do anything moving forward. forward. However, the Alcoholics Anonymous/Narcotics Anonymous program teaches you to remain present, focusing on one day, one moment at a time. After 34 years clean and sober, my life has never been better. My sobriety has brought me everything that I could possibly wish for.

Elton John

I'm very happy I'm an alcoholic – it's a great gift, because wherever I go, the abyss follows me. It's a volcanic anger you have, and it's fuel. Rocket fuel. But of course it can rip you to pieces and kill you.

Anthony Hopkins

I know I've got a reputation that I'm this depressed guy. I'm not — I'm a happy guy. But I went through some really dark patches and I drank my way through them. I couldn't be as good as I wanted to be. It drove me crazy. The drinking was part of it. If I couldn't be as good as I wanted to be, I'd just drown it with booze. It was a way to numb out, to not feel what I was feeling.

Billy Joel

I had a great drinking career, and I'm retired from it now. I just went cold turkey. Seeing the results that come from it, and my psychology around it, it made it easy to sacrifice what I wanted in order to get where I want. I was at a point in my life where I was ready to engineer my choices around my end result. Nothing tastes better than feeling really good, being able to do things, and having a clear mindset.

Zac Brown

On Jan. 4, 2016, then-Atlanta Falcons coaches Quinn, Kyle Shanahan and Raheem Morris all sat me down and told me they believed I was drinking too often. I agreed with them. I had to relay that message to my wife, Katie, and her look of disappointment drove me to change my life. It was that moment that I said, 'I will never drink again.' I've been sober since that day.

Mike McDaniel

I remember when I first got sober and all the shit was out of my system. I couldn't picture myself being able to do anything without some kind of drug. But I remember just being, like, really happy and everything was fucking new to me again. I feel like all the years that I was using, I wasn't growing as a person. I started treating sobriety like a superpower.

Eminem

If we're not measuring it by how much we drink but how we perform as a human being—then I would say alcohol is a problem for me because I'm not at my best. I've found that life keeps happening regardless of whether I'm sober or not, but today I get to show up for it. I like showing up 100%, 100% of the time. I love that if anything comes in an opportunity, I can say yes knowing that I'm going to be ready. I don't have to get ready. It's been really important for me over the last year living a sober lifestyle, because I really wanted to polish up my craft.

Miley Cyrus

I don't drink.

Tom Cruise

I got sober. I stopped killing myself with alcohol. I began to think: 'Wait a minute - if I can stop doing this, what are the possibilities?' It seemed that I performed better sober than drunk. Who knew?

Craig Ferguson

The reason I don't drink is because my gift is tied squarely to my mental alertness and sharpness. Once you alter your mental state you immediately start to diminish your gift.

Steve Harvey

I've seen so many brilliant children of brilliant people go bad and become tremendous failures. And I find that so much of it is caused by drugs, alcohol, you know, different substances. And I always would say to my kids, 'No drugs, no alcohol, no cigarettes.'

Donald Trump

I'm sober and want nothing back from my old life. Success is the warmest place to hide. When you're so proud that you won't change, you've got problems.

Terry Crews

Alcohol, drugs and nicotine were getting in the way. I was relying on a source outside of myself to create, and that's not authentic, because you're not yourself. Where I am now, sobriety is serving me, and I'm creating from a different place, It's coming from me, it's not coming from liquor, it's not coming from a party environment.

Doechii

There are women succeeding beyond their wildest dreams because of their sobriety.

Marry Karr

6. Quotes on the Family Side

Marriage, Parenting, Relatives, Relationships

If I were not a parent, I am fairly certain that I would still be a heavy drinker today. In 2017, my day began with sending my kids off to school and heading to the office — usually with a mild hangover. Around dinnertime I'd pour my first glass of Cabernet, and once my little ones were in bed, it was certain I'd finish the rest of the bottle. I couldn't drink the way I wanted to drink and parent the way I wanted to parent. And that for me ultimately—it came down to a choice.

Celeste Yvonne

We can't expect to keep beer in the refrigerator and expect our fifteen-year-old not to drink beer. We have an impact on our children by what we say, but particularly by what we do. They forget many of the things we say, but they observe everything we do.

Truett Cathy

Nope. Don't drink. I used to drink. When we had kids and my kids were growing up, I decided I didn't want to set that kind of example for them, so I just quit drinking and it's probably the best thing I ever did. Never have a hangover, never feel bad. I just don't do it. You have more fun and you enjoy [life] more. You enjoy the relationships more. It's been a good thing for me, one of the best things I've decided to do.

Nick Saban

No hangovers, no regret, no wasted time—just living fully in the moment. There's just no better gift. There's no better gift I can give my kids; there's no better gift I can give my husband.

Jessica Simpson

My problem was not only drinking; it was selfishness. The booze was leading me to put myself ahead of others, especially my family. I loved Laura and the girls too much to let that happen. I do know that I have a habitual personality. I was drinking too much, and it was starting to create problems. Alcohol can compete with your affections. It sure did in my case — affections with your family, or affections for exercise. It was the competition that I decided just wasn't worth it. As a matter of fact, I don't think I would've quit drinking had it not been for being a dad.

George W. Bush

Two months before my child was born, I was just drinking a lot. Cherry said, 'If my waters break, do you really want someone else to drive me to the hospital?' That was it. I realized I didn't want to miss that moment — or be holding my child drunk. I quit drinking for my daughter. It all came at the same time of wanting to be a responsible dad, wanting to feel and look good.

Ed Sheeran

As a business owner and a father, even if you didn't drink all week and then Friday night you had a few, I would wake up Saturday morning and just be tired and not engaged with my kids as much as I wanted to.

Colin Plume.

I really wasn't able to enjoy parenting when I'd been drinking the night before. My girls were the ultimate motivation to stop. They were six months and two when I stopped. And now nearly four and five and they'll have no memory of me drinking. Sobriety has also allowed me to rebuild and strengthen my relationships. I'm more present with my loved ones, more empathetic, and more honest – both with myself and others. Alcohol took away my joy and made it harder to show up as the mum and partner I wanted to be.

Millie Mackintosh

The cure for addiction is suffering. You suffer enough that something inside you goes, 'I'm done.' And I'm lucky, because I hit that point before I lost really the things that were the most important. It was not my career or money — it was my relationship with my kids. When I felt as if it impacted them, I recognized it. It was the worst day of my life.

Ben Affleck

I knew it was affecting my personal relationships. It was affecting my professional relationships. It was affecting my family. It was turning me into a person that I didn't want to be. I knew I was at a point where I could lose everything in my life. First and foremost, my family.

Tim McGraw

I realized I was losing these special moments with my loved ones and that I had been constantly missing out due to my drinking addiction.

Kevin Kreider

I really did it for my son Conor, because I thought, no matter what kind of human being I was, I couldn't stand being around him like that. I couldn't bear the idea that, as he experienced enough of life to form a picture of me, it would be a picture of the man I was then.

Eric Clapton

On Jan. 4, 2016, then-Atlanta Falcons coaches Quinn, Kyle Shanahan and Raheem Morris all sat me down and told me they believed I was drinking too often. I agreed with them. I had to relay that message to my wife, Katie, and her look of disappointment drove me to change my life. It was that moment that I said, 'I will never drink again.' I've been sober since that day.

Mike McDaniel

As I got older and was raising kids, I could definitely start to see that my disease was starting to progress. I was drinking and driving. I was drinking and driving with my kids in the car. My husband had moved out of our family home, and it was because of the alcohol. My kids were upstairs sleeping, and I was drinking downstairs. I wasn't a safe mom at that time.

Carrie Bates

There's addiction in my family and I've chosen to not drink. I am a real outsider in my family. At a very young age I announced to everyone that I was never going to drink. It probably felt like a betrayal of my family and their entire legacy, but I have stuck to it. I come from a beer family and I've never had a drink.

Gillian Jacobs

I just couldn't see the light. And I had these two kids that I had to fight for and be the best person, and they always inspired me to be my best.

Drew Barrymore

I lost seven years of my life to alcohol use disorder before I finally got sober. I was too drunk or hungover to show up for the people I cared about.

Gregory Gourdet

The greatest gift of being free from drugs and alcohol is being a part of my family again. Life for me is more important than alcohol.

Oksana Baiul

The kids knew; Dakota and Stella called me on it. I am from an alcoholic family and I know how consuming the struggle can be It's not something that you choose, it's genetic and it's really strong. You just can't get enough. Your own will cannot stop it. I think part of the reason my marriage to Antonio fell apart was because I was stuck; nobody else is to blame. It's just that I personally got stuck and I won't let that happen again.

Melanie Griffith

My relationship with my kids is much better since I got sober. I'm a much more connected and present parent, which is amazing. Pretty much every aspect of my life has changed as a result of my sobriety.

Lily Allen

Yesterday my son turned eight. Which means that I haven't had a drink for eight years and eight months. And I have handled my business day in and day out without booze. I got sober when I was twenty-five. I figured out early on that the most important parts of life, for me, would be sobriety, relationships, love, and faith.

Glennon Doyle

I had to quit drinking. I mean it was just not doing anything good for me and it ends by going to dark places in my family and the whole thing. Substance abuse is the top predictor of marital breakdown and long-term unhappiness.

Arthur Brooks

I'm not sure Steve and I would have made it long enough to have Ellen and Charlie had I not been sober and trying to live an authentic, honest life rather than trying to outrun, outsmart, and numb vulnerability. As much as I try to work a 'live and let live' vibe, I've watched 'civilized drinking' ravage the lives of so many families and friends that I've developed no interest in it at all.

Brené Brown

Alcoholism doesn't just run, it sprints in our family. I don't do just one drink. I commend your ability to really just have one drink… I wish I had that. 4. I have an addictive personality.

Logan Paul

I think the scariest addiction on this planet is to alcohol. It ruins families, it ruins relationships. I've told my kids about that: 'You've got the crazy gene in you, guys. When it comes time to kick back with the buddies, drink a beer, and watch a football game, just realize that there will be a day when that thing turns on you. So you better keep an eye on it.

Nikki Sixx

I'm so proud that our kids will never ever see me intoxicated. I'm so proud that I have built a life that feels not boring.

Abby Wambach

I came from a broken situation. My father was an alcoholic and he beat the crap out of me and told me I would never amount to nothing, so my pain led me to my greatness and my greatness led me to my destructive behavior. I'm not unique. I'm a recovering addict just like millions. Beer was the foundation of our alcoholic lifestyle. I was achieving great things on the outside, but on the inside, I was empty. I was broken. You have to allow yourself to be healed on the inside from that brokenness.

Darryl Strawberry

Many people ask me why I never drink alcohol. I tell them it's because when I was young I watched it destroy my father. When my father was alive, I once picked up his bottle and tried to drink from it. He rushed to stop me and told me it was poison for children, so I asked him why he drank it himself.

Cristiano Ronaldo

My kids even came to a few therapy sessions with me. And that was especially important, because they got to kind of let loose, telling me how my addiction affected them, too. We were struggling. That's what keeps me sober, because I missed so much time with my kids because of my career and then my extracurricular activity when I wasn't playing. My children were really happy that I went through the recovery process. I was thinking a lot, too much, about how they would think of me, but once I let down that guard, let them in and let them know everything I was going through, I think it helped build our relationship.

Lamar Odom

It was years of waking up in the morning and seeing my wife crying, which let me know that I had fucked up the night before. Now I haven't had a drink in almost 14 years. I wanted my mother and father to see their son sober again before they left this earth for good.

Sugar Ray Leonard

I put my wife through a lot in our marriage and she's a very strong woman. It's about time I became the strong one in the relationship, take responsibility and take the lead in making choices, making decisions and stepping up and being the man I'm supposed to be and not continue to hurt her, put my kids in situations where they might hear things. It's not a good situation for anybody. When you're doing this, you don't mean to hurt anybody, but you're only thinking it hurts yourself, but I know it hurt a lot of people.

Josh Hamilton

I can't think of one thing that drinking has done that's been good for me or my family. I knew I had a problem. It was what I did when I drank, the choices I made. I once said, 'I am not drinking anymore.' My wife said, 'I don't want to hear it. I've heard it so many times.' And I said, 'You're right. I'm gonna go to rehab.' I went to please her and to show everyone that I was serious. I admitted my problem, I was in there for 28 days, and it worked.

Brett Favre

Alcoholism runs in my family. So, for me, I knew it was something that was always a crutch. I always knew I had a problem. I feel like I was screaming down a dark hallway and everyone's like, 'Figure it out.' I put my fiancée through hell and nobody knew… nobody believed her.

Maxx Crosby

My mom died with a broken heart. Her dying wish was for me to get sober. I didn't give it to her, and that haunts me.

Chris Herren

Fear was a big motivator for me. Losing my family, that was the thing that scared me so much, that was the bottom I hit. My wife kicked me out of the house. She said, 'You've got to go somewhere and sort this shit out.' I realized if I didn't seek help, I could lose my family. I entered rehab and basically had to be torn down to bones. Seven weeks of ripping your life apart, anything you thought you had – gone – then rebuilding it sober.

James Hetfield

My mom asked me not to drink alcohol. I loved my mom so much and I wanted to do that for her. That's why I didn't drink. I built a huge part of my life around wine, but I don't need alcohol to be happy for one second.

Gary Vaynerchuk

It took me a long time to get sober. Took me a long time to recognize my alcoholism. I didn't drink like my dad, so I compared everything to him. it just took a long time for me. In 2006, my wife called an intervention on me. I knew that was it. I'm like, 'Oh, this is that fork in the road. Here it is.' I had to learn a different way to be in the world without drugs and alcohol. It's a lot to do with my dad and being born into a family with an alcoholic father. My job is to now maybe break that chain and do something different.

Keith Urban

I want my kids to look at me and know I'm gonna do whatever I say I gonna do. I want them to know they can trust me, that I'm gonna be reliable. I was doing things I wasn't enjoying and didn't want to be doing.

Theo Von

Sixteen years sober and never looking back I've been sober since the accident, but I've replaced all of my bad addictions with good ones. I gave up on smoking, drinking and doing drugs years ago. I went from being addicted to drugs, to being addicted to spending time with my kids now.

Travis Barker

My dad died of alcoholism. My dad stone-cold drank himself to oblivion. Cirrhosis of the liver. He died July 3, 1998. And that always hung over my head. I never took it lightly that that was in my sphere of influence. I've got teenage kids, and they need to see a sober dad.

Ben Harper

The catalyst was Amanda Shires, who's my wife now. I was trying to establish a long-term relationship with her, and it became pretty clear to me that she wasn't going to be in a long-term relationship with a drunk. So that was my first real motivation to get sober. I don't think I would have done it—I certainly wouldn't have done it at that point— if it hadn't been for her. She called a bunch of people that were my friends and whose opinions I respected—it took a lot of courage and care on her part—and figured out how to get me into rehab.

Jason Isbell

As I have reflected on my father's influence in my life, one of the things I am most grateful for is that he chose not to drink any alcohol. It would have been fine if he did, but his abstinence was a powerful example for me, maybe even more than he realized at the time. Kids imitate their father's behaviors and therefore, I encourage fathers to be careful with alcohol, and don't get near anything else that's mind altering. It's just not worth being part of the crowd in that way, and the downside may be far worse than the upside could ever be for you and your sons.

Tony Dungy

My life has turned around. I found the other half of me, which was my wife. I reconnected with my children, who wouldn't come near me. I said sorry to everybody I could find—some of them said, "Okay"; some of them said, "Go away." Alcohol ate a hole in me where loving and caring had been. But all of that came back.

Joe Walsh

I am a raging alcoholic and a raging addict and I didn't want to see my kids do the same thing. You realize the kids have got this fear in their eyes. I mean, it's a very selfish disease. My kids needed me.

Ozzy Osbourne

Everything is magnified when you have a child with special needs. James was about 2 when I got sober, and he was a big, big part of me putting the bottle down. I was in no position to be a father to a child like him. if it wasn't for my sobriety, I wouldn't be able to be there for James and enjoy the marvel of his life and support him in the way that I feel that I can.

Colin Farrell

I never could have imagined this. I sit right here and think how it could have turned out so differently. I was a functioning alcoholic. I thought all serious artists were self-destructive. That anybody worth their salt was going to be out there living on the edge. I never thought I'd live past 30. I could have ended up dead. At the time I just went cold turkey. I didn't want to die before my daughter grew up.

Kris Kristofferson

Being over five years sober feels like a real milestone in my life. I don't judge other people's drinking; I just know it doesn't fit the life and parent I want to be. It's just the way I do it — which I personally think is really fun and awesome — is just not the kind of fun and awesome that goes with having a child for me. When I'm at a stage in my life where there is enough space for me to have a hangover, I'll start drinking again, but that won't be until my kid is out of the house. I'm not drinking while my son lives at home, because I don't like how I drink and he needs me in the mornings.

Anne Hathaway

When I finally stopped, it was because my life was turning professional, I was getting married, planning to have kids, and I could see alcohol did not fit that future. I decided to abstain completely; for a long time I was disgusted by alcohol and felt it just poisoned and polluted people. All I see is that alcohol makes drinkers stupid and fuzzy minded, even though they feel cool.

Jordan Peterson

I was a blackout drinker: I would wake up in places and not know how I got there. In 1991, my wife and daughter found me passed out in the kitchen... The next day, I was in rehab. The most valuable thing I have is my sobriety. Because without that, I don't have anything.

Samuel L. Jackson

I admit I struggled with alcohol and it weighed heavily on me. It was self-inflicted, but when Tawanna divorced me, that's when I knew I hit my lowest point and it was time for some deep, self-re-evaluation. I had to change a lot of things. I had to convince her that basically this wasn't the same old me. Ultimately, when you evaluate your maturation and what's important and what you mean to your family and friends and the world, I just thought about the way I was supposed to be in life. And I didn't see how alcohol was helping any. All I could think about was negative experiences. I realized alcohol was a big problem, and I was tired of fighting it.

Allen Iverson

Many people ask me why I never drink alcohol. I tell them it's because when I was young I watched it destroy my father. When my father was alive, I once picked up his bottle and tried to drink from it. He rushed to stop me and told me it was poison for children, so I asked him why he drank it himself.

Cristiano Ronaldo

Above anything else—above family or job—the main thing is staying sober. That's because without being sober, I don't have a family or a job.

William Regal

I wouldn't give a nanosecond's worth of thought to die for my children, to kill for my children. But I couldn't stop drinking for my children. Alcohol robbed me of the ability to see others. Getting sober was the single bravest thing I've ever done, and will ever do, in my life. Being courageous enough to acknowledge it privately with my family and friends.

Elizabeth Vargas

One morning I'd forgotten my daughter had an appointment I'd promised to drive her to, and I'd already had a couple of pops that day. So had to call my friend Tony to take us. We got her there on time, but it broke my heart because she was in the backseat and I could just tell she was thinking, 'Why isn't dad driving?' So I got home and sat with that for the rest of the day.

Charlie Sheen

My mother fell off the wagon at my rehearsal dinner. Shortly after that, she got sober and was sober until she died, almost 80, so more than 20 years. I was in my early 30s, and it's almost like she got sober right about the time my drinking picked up. I say it's almost like our genetic code owed the universe some really wretched alcoholic, and I stepped into the slot as she left it.

Mary Karr

I remember like it was yesterday: My mom telling me on the answering machine to 'pick up, pick up' because my grandpa had had a heart attack. I couldn't deal with it in the state I was in, and I needed to go to sleep to wake up so I could deal with it. Who doesn't keep a bottle of Cuervo Gold by their bedside table? That was the final wake-up call. I've been sober ever since.

Rob Lowe

I was lost. I was hiding and doing what people who drink too much do. I was not connecting. I used to live an isolated existence, even in relationships, but now my family knows me for who I really am.

Tim Allen

My mother said to me when I was 59, she said, 'Denzel, you do a lot of good. You have to do good the right way and you know what I'm talking about.' I don't drink anymore. I made a commitment to completely cut out drinking and anything that might hamper me from getting my mind and body together.

Denzel Washington

I had a brother, Fred. He had a problem with alcohol, and he would tell me, 'Don't drink. Don't drink.' He was substantially older, and I listened to him. From the time my kids could practically speak, I would say that: 'No drugs, no alcohol, no smoking.' And if you never start them, it's so easy. If you don't start it, you don't have a longing.

Donald Trump

I'm not a drinker. I'm the only Irish man you've ever met who's never had a drink. I remember taking out a fifth of, I think it was gin, and put it on the kitchen table. But I couldn't even make myself take a drink. What saved me was really my boys. There are enough alcoholics in my family.

Joe Biden

I was afraid that I wouldn't be able to work anymore if I quit drinking and drugging, but I decided (again, so far as I was able to decide anything in my distraught and depressed state of mind) that I would trade writing for staying married and watching the kids grow up.

Stephen King

7. Quotes on the Lifestyle Side

Habits, Interests, Sobriety, Leisure, Freedom

In quitting, I didn't lose anything. In quitting, I learned how to be the person I wanted to be. When people ask me when I knew it was time to quit drinking, I often say: when the shame of my drinking became louder than the relief it gave me. I decided that I didn't want to moderate; I wanted to quit drinking altogether. Today I am at peace knowing I will never drink again. I am happy, giddy even, knowing alcohol will not control me anymore. I used to drink to numb my brain, my heart, my feelings. Now I feel everything, and recognize what my body is trying to tell me. I will never drink again. I don't ever want to drink again.

Celeste Yvonne

Sobriety has given me everything I value — my family, my career, and my health. Without it, I'd have nothing. We put way too much energy and effort into the worst day and we forget the first day. Sobriety has made me better at everything in my life.. I think it's about self-worth. I think it's about confidence and self-esteem. I think it's about family. It's about the people that love you. I'm unbelievably grateful. I have to pinch myself for the life it's given me. Sobriety will enable you to become the man you always wanted to be. You will find your life's purpose from your struggles.

Chris Herren

I feel like a different person now that I'm sober. Twelve years ago when I quit drinking, I stopped going out to bars and doing things like that. I wouldn't trade these 12 years for nothing. I'm at peace. When I played golf before, I realized the only reason I wanted to play was to drink. After a while, instead of thinking, 'How many beers can we drink in 18 holes?' I fell into a pattern of what could I do to get good at golf. I realized with each passing day I really didn't like drinking.

Brett Favre

I lived the majority of my adult life sober. I was great sober. The problem was, when I did have a drink, I couldn't stop. There were no brakes. When you don't have an off switch, you go until you can't go anymore. I fully identify as an addict alcoholic. I think my whole nature is really all or nothing. I have two speeds: go and go faster. Part of being sober is I don't want to miss a moment of life, of that texture, even if that means being in some pain.

Demi Moore

I quit because I was finally fed up and disgusted by how much alcohol had taken over my life. Thirty-three years ago I found recovery and a tribe that has sustained me on my incredible, grateful journey. My life is full of love, family, God, opportunity friends work, dogs and fun.

Rob Lowe

When you stop drinking, your life becomes way less exciting. There's a lot of boredom and maybe some insecurity that you're not doing enough interesting things. But if you stick with that feeling long enough, you start to find out what you actually truly enjoy. And when you focus on those things, there is a quiet satisfaction that takes over. Quitting alcohol is completely reshaped my definition of pleasure, enjoyment, and fun. And because I no longer crave constant novelty and stimulation, it's actually been much easier to be consistent with my actions. I've developed habits in this past year that I've always wanted, but I've never been able to manage throughout my life. Exercise habits that I struggled to create for years have suddenly fallen into place, and my food choices are far more conscious and less compulsive than they were before. I don't have these maddening cravings for junk food in the middle of the night, and I certainly don't have to deal with the drunk munchies.

Mark Manson

As long as I don't drink I am living my best life. Alcohol was running my life long before I admitted it. I know this about myself, and it was very hard to come to grips with it. And I drank right through till I was 34. One day I just said, 'You've had too much fun,' and I quit and I haven't had anything to drink in 36 years. I forget now that I even ever drank, it's been so long. I don't feel like I miss much. It's so nice to have your control back.

David Letterman

Now I feel free. I don't drink. I don't take pills. Nothing. I am most grateful. And it's fantastic. It's like getting out of prison.

Melanie Griffith

I used to drink. Yes, I did. The truth is the truth. And after I had fought and beat somebody, I didn't hardly go nowhere without two big, pretty women beside me. But my change is one of the things that will mark me as a great man in history. When you can live righteous in the hell of North America—when a man can control his life, his physical needs, his lower self, he elevates himself.

Muhammad Ali

If you need booze or drugs to enjoy your life to the fullest you are doing it wrong. I was an alcoholic – a drunk – even when I told myself I just had 'a little problem with alcohol.' I just want to take it easy now. This is good news. It's the whole thing of taking it slow. And it's so much better. I am happier, and not afraid to be unhappy. That's OK too. And then you can be like, all is good. And that is the thing, that is the gift.

Robin Williams

I just wanted to do dry January and all I could think about was having a drink. I couldn't quite wrap my head around how much I was struggling without booze in that first month — and It really scared me. I decided, as a sort of punishment to myself, that I would do February as well as January. If I can do two months off then I can prove to myself that I don't have a problem. Two months go by and I was still really struggling. I decided that I would wait until my birthday, which is June 1st. I said to myself if I can do six months without alcohol then I can prove to myself that I don't have a problem. And by the time I had got to June 1st I was the happiest I'd ever been in my life. I could sleep better, I could handle problems better, things that would go wrong on set that would normally set me off I could take in my stride. I had so much such better mental clarity. I felt healthier I felt fitter. By the time I'd crossed that annual mark I was done. I was like, 'I'm never gonna drink again because this is the best version of myself.'

Tom Holland

What I see in so many people that recover successfully, they become passionate about something. Like writing music, or painting, or hiking, or, like, building ships in bottles. It doesn't matter what it is, but it's, like, a highly specified thing, and it either gives you a respite from the world or it gives you a creative outlet and it occupies your mind in a productive way. I like myself and my life so much more now.

Julien Baker

There's nothing beneficial about consuming alcohol. If you really don't need to drink, then don't. Find another hobby. Don't waste your time. You're better than that. Try hot air ballooning.

Tom Segura

It's hard in the early days because there isn't a prize when you stop drinking... quitting a substance you're physically and emotionally addicted to often leaves you even more vulnerable at first. Just know that it's going to be hard, and that you have to lean in to the pain, because that's where you'll find the answers, and eventually the light. Sobriety has given me my life. It has given me my authentic self for the first time. Strangely, life now is no less intense than it was when I was partying hard in my early 20s, it's just more authentic, and more productive. Whether I like where my life goes or not, I know that alcohol isn't steering the ship. It's all me, for better or for worse.

Hayley Gibson

Rather than viewing a brief relapse back to inactivity as a failure, treat is as a challenge and try to get back on track as soon as possible. Life is a series of relapses and recoveries

Jimmy Connors

Unlike many people who quit, I've never wanted to drink again. Once I got past the first six months, I just felt so much better. I was so grateful. I've enjoyed being sober a lot, and that's a huge blessing. It's not like I have an especially strong character. I don't. If you put a tray of Fig Newtons right here, you would see how weak I really am. It's just on this one thing—the booze and drugs—it's like, I don't want that at all.

Tucker Carlson

I quit drinking after someone close to me challenged me to go sober for a month. Well, a month turned into two decades of living the sober life. It has just made my life so much more simplified. I certainly didn't need alcohol in my life kind of muddying up my weekends. And so I removed that factor entirely, and it certainly has made my life better.

Amber Mac

I'm just a better person when I don't drink, in every area of my life. It is 10 years since I used drugs or drank alcohol and my life has improved immeasurably. I have a job, a house, a cat, good friendships and generally a bright outlook.

Russell Brand

There are setbacks... there's times you move forward and do great, and there's times you set back. And that'll probably be a process throughout the rest of my life and something that I have to be diligent about.

Tim McGraw

I thought I had everything under control. I would start going through cycles where I'd try to stop cold turkey. It would always be two or three months sober, then a relapse. I would make rules for myself: 'I'm only going to drink wine' or 'I'm only going to drink beer'... but I could never stick to them. Getting sober six years ago definitely gave me some clarity. I always tell people, if you think you might have a problem, you probably have a problem. It took me 28 years to realize that I had a problem. People always talk about sobriety and say everything is better, but I can attest that it really is. There is NOTHING that I am more grateful for than my sobriety. Without that being my number one, everything else would disappear.

CC Sabathia

Elite athletes aren't easy people to get sober. We have pretty big egos, usually. I talk about recovery openly. I was sick of getting A's in Treatment and F's in Life. I lost everything in my drinking, except my life. The only thing I didn't lose was my life. The number one reason people don't get help is not financial. It is shame. Sobriety was the hardest thing I've ever done. It was way harder than winning an Olympic gold medal. It's so much bigger than the medals. There's not a part of my life that sobriety hasn't changed.

Carrie Bates

Not having a drink for over a year and a half, it's incredible. It's not only my body — on a lot of different levels. It's been amazing. I go to bed earlier. I sleep more. I wake up every day and have a completely clear head. I don't feel like my head went through a brick wall. There are so many positives to it.

Michael Phelps

Incorporating diet, exercise, and mental health therapy into my daily routine helped me maintain sobriety. Physical fitness goals, such as preparing for 'Baywatch,' motivated healthy living while therapy provided essential mental health support to sustain my recovery.

Zac Efron

The first thing I did, I stopped going to bars for six months. Within that first year I would go running — I would literally go run at night after work instead of going out drinking. Last week I marked 14 years clean, sober and smoke free. I'm not afraid of alcohol. It doesn't dictate my life. I know who I am, and alcohol no longer defines me. I had to make a clear decision. I just wanted more, and I deserved more, and I could achieve more. I want to be sober for the rest of my life — that's something I work at every day.

Gregory Gourdet

Ultrarunners can't be alcoholics, can they? I'm proof alcoholics can hide in plain sight. I was so enslaved by drink I swigged wine during an ultra-marathon. For almost 25 years I was a functioning alcoholic. I drank pretty much every single day. And not just a pint at lunchtime. We are talking bottles and bottles of wine, beer, whatever was there.

I was drinking to the point of blackout at least once a week. When I got sober, I had to do a lot of work on myself. I used my values (kindness, honesty and integrity) as a guideline for this, and I still use them every single day. The booze anxiety had been replaced by a desperate need to help people – to make up for what I had done in some way. I burn 75% brighter since I stopped drinking.

Allie Bailey

I feel better not drinking. Living with integrity and living in control of my own self, that's the life I want now. It's more fun. I have such a desire to want to keep this feeling and stay this way, and I'm willing to do whatever it takes. I'm in a different headspace. I don't want those things I wanted before.

Lindsay Lohan

I love my life. I have nothing but gratitude. Somebody said if you're going to do things that you have to say you're sorry for tomorrow, don't do it. So I don't do things like that. It's moment by moment. I'm 68 percent joyous, aiming for 70 percent. And I'm extremely grateful for where I am today.

Tim Allen

I was a really voracious reader in my teens and that was one of the things I found drinking took away from me, bizarrely, as a side effect. I didn't have the compulsion or energy to read anything. So I've got that back.

Daniel Radcliffe

I'm sober and loving life. I used to b happy when I was high. Now I'm happy when I'm sober. No judgement to anyone. Be gentle with yourself.

Nicki Minaj

Since opening my own modelling agency, I take care of myself now. I feel like I've grown up. I used to be a night person but now I go to bed at 11 pm and get up at 8 am. I like to start my day with tea and meditation, followed by some Pilates or yoga. I'm a bit groggy in the afternoon if I don't get eight hours sleep. I don't really go to clubs anymore. I'm actually quite settled. Living in Highgate with my dog and my husband and my daughter! I don't want to go back to how I was.

Kate Moss

I was a highly functioning alcoholic. Alcohol was a daily occurrence, big time, all day long. Then I would come home and take four Excedrin and drink a giant liter of water to combat the headache and hangover the next day. I would get in a hot bathtub and often fall asleep. Now I don't drink, I don't smoke, I don't do drugs. I drink caffeine, I play tennis, I take care of my son. I have no desire to have a drink whatsoever. It's very interesting. Absolutely none. I am much happier not drinking. And no, I do not sip wine with dinner. Not a smart thing for an alcoholic to do!

Tom Ford

I'd come to a point in my life where I just felt like I'd had enough. I was determined never to have another hangover in my life because they are such a waste of time. I didn't like the way it made me feel anymore. I just wanted to be present. I thought I'd be boring or that I wouldn't be able to dance or have fun, but it's actually the opposite. I feel more confident because I'm fully there. Since I stopped drinking, my creative channels have opened up in a way I didn't expect. I'm much more consistent as a person, as a mother, as a friend.

Sarah Jane Clarke

In the end, I just thought I didn't want the life I had. I didn't like the person I was. I hated the person I saw in the mirror. I am 22 years sober today. I sometimes think of my life as before and after. Alcohol is cunning, baffling—the disease of addiction is cunning, baffling, and powerful. Most people did not know anything about my struggle with a brain disease. And I'm so grateful to be here today.

Kathryn Burgum

Being sober has given me a gift that I didn't know I needed: freedom. Freedom to be myself, freedom to be the mother I want to be and that my daughters deserve, freedom to be an introvert, freedom to be healthy, and freedom not to mask any part of me with a manufactured air of confidence. Anything in your life that is making you unhappy, whether it's alcohol, whether it's a person, whatever it is – that toxic habit. Don't wait to change. Just do it because you never know how long you've got left. Life is short and if something is stealing your joy, make the change. Sobriety has been the ultimate act of self-love. It has been messy and hard and uncomfortable at times but it has transformed me in ways I never thought possible.

Millie Mackintosh

Instead of going to drink, I started finding other things, like just being comfortable in your own skin and being okay. I am sober and grateful. Sobriety was the best gift I ever gave myself. Before, I was at war with myself and I didn't want to admit it. The greatest gift of being free from drugs and alcohol is being a part of my family again. Life for me is more important than alcohol. I've gone from alcoholic to workaholic.

Oksana Baiul

To feel so free and able day in day out, is a true joy! If you'd told me I would toast my 40th birthday with a glass of water, I'd have thought you were crackers. When I decided to go sober, I never knew how long it would last. Sobriety didn't magically fix my life — it gave me the chance to face it. I hid behind booze for so so so many years of my life. Now I fly free, and I've never ever, ever felt better! My life is the clearest, happiest, it's precious to me, REALLY precious, to have the clarity.

Lisa Riley

Today, this right here is happiness. I don't drink or party anymore. Clubs are no longer my scene. I can be around other people while they drink, but I don't want it. These days I stay sober with routine. I work out every day, try to eat right and drink a lot of water, and I make time to take care of myself. Once I realized what my future held if I didn't change, I found the strength to move forward. For a long, long time, the only thing that would help me put a smile on my face is if I was drinking. But I eventually realized that's not happiness.

Mary J. Blige

I had to lose everything—my marriage, my money, and my self-respect—before I was willing to change. We all deserve a second chance, but we have to be willing to do the work to earn it. I realized this life was a gift I needed to prize like nothing I had ever prized before. Within six months of breaking my addiction, at age 31, I was breaking masters world records. Swimming was my sanctuary, but sobriety was my salvation.

Karlyn Pipes

Sobriety has just changed my life immeasurably. My life has never been as fulfilling as it is now. Everything is going well, and I believe that wouldn't be the case if I weren't sober. I think I'm just a completely different person. I don't think I'd be married to my husband. I don't think that my kids would be thriving in the way that they are. I don't think that I'd have gone into finding acting and how much I enjoy that. I definitely wouldn't be getting as much sleep. I go to the gym four times a week. Pretty much every aspect of my life has changed as a result of my sobriety. I actually don't even know if I'd be alive if I'm honest if I hadn't got sober. So yeah, that's definitely at the top of my gratitude list when I go to bed every night is my sobriety.

Lily Allen

Sobriety, if it is anything, is paying attention, seeing the wonder and the beauty around us that we so easily sprint by. This is actually living. My passage into sobriety was both slow and fast. Slow, in that it took me seventeen years to realize alcohol had never done me any favors. But now I can say with certainty, I'll never have a drink again. I don't want to. Alcohol is just a cheap substitute for real life. For me, going home sober at the end of the night and waking up without a hangover felt like the most wonderfully delicious thing I'd ever experienced.

Holly Whitaker

Life still happens after you stop drinking. You don't get sober and then all your anxiety vanishes and depression vanishes and life challenges vanish and trauma and tragedy vanish. Recovery is something you deal with on a daily basis. There is no such thing as you're all clear and you don't have to work on this any longer. Drinking to escape was profoundly selfish, and all those unresolved resentments and worries metastasized while I drank to ignore them.

Elizabeth Vargas

You cannot feel better than having a fit body and the resilient, healthy mind that goes with it. One of the considerable advantages of not drinking is the improved quality of life as your broken sleeping patterns repair and you begin to catch up on the lost sleep. This will have a phenomenal impact on your quality of life. Waking up feeling fresh and ready to go is one of the great feelings in life. When you stop drinking, life becomes immeasurably better, but it is still life, with all its ups and downs. Over the years my drinking steadily increased. I knew for a fact that if I stopped for long enough I would start to feel much better. In February 2014, I finally stopped for good.

William Porter

When I first quit drinking, nine years ago, I thought I'd be giving up fun, spontaneity, holidays, parties. Instead, I gave up hangovers, 3 a.m. shame, and the constant anxiety about how much I'd drunk. Now my life is so much better and more rewarding without it, I can't imagine going back there. I'm much more positive about life, which makes me a much easier person to live with. One of the best gifts of sobriety is peace. Going sober has transformed my life.

Clare Pooley

Sobriety just feels like... Nothing. I wake up in the morning and it's Nothing. I leave the house and walk to my intended destination feeling Nothing. Nothingness is peaking. Nothing is luxurious. And Nothing is meditative. When I first got sober, my biggest reservation was that I was terrified of becoming boring. Once I removed the substances, I was able to see how incredibly unpredictable, how incredibly un-boring, life can be.

Cat Marnell

Getting and staying sober was the hardest work I'd ever done. I didn't love it at first. I thought maybe there would be some loopholes in the basic premise of abstinence... It turned out that there were no loopholes. Being sober delivered almost everything drinking promised. I've never had a hangover in these past 37 years, and I've never done anything that I was ashamed of the next day, which is a pretty incredible trade-off. Sobriety gave me everything alcohol and drugs promised—belonging, self-respect, more laughter than you can even imagine, and profound companionship.

Anne Lamott

To rediscover joy in sobriety is an amazing thing. It's the emotional equivalent of realizing that your shoes are painfully tight and then sighing with relief when you finally take them off. There's something about sober living and sober thinking, about facing long afternoons without the numbing distraction of anesthesia, that disabuses you of the belief in externals, shows you that strength and hope come not from circumstances or the acquisition of things but from the simple accumulation of active experience, from gritting the teeth and checking the items off the list, one by one, even though it's painful and you're afraid.

Caroline Knapp

Finally, I got sober. I gave up drinking, and it was a new beginning. Removing alcohol was one of the best decisions I have made in my adult life. And this is me today: drinking Perrier, not wine; clear-eyed, writing this morning, celebrating 15 years of serenity, happy in my skin, and forever grateful to the many who supported me on this journey, above all Nicholas, my son.

Ann Dowsett Johnston

What I didn't know was how terribly high the price was going to be. It was going to cost me friends, familial love, many boyfriends, the respect of my colleagues and all of my self esteem. Crushing hangovers turn even the simplest tasks – taking a cheque to the bank or buying food for dinner – into arduous nightmares. Sober, I felt free! My world got bigger. I discovered that I was about a million times happier sober than I ever had been while drinking. I found myself with dozens more hours in the week, heaps more energy, more money, deepened friendships, revived family relationships, better skin, a tighter body, tanned legs for the first time ever, the ability to sleep for eight uninterrupted hours, a bone deep sense of well-being, a totally turned around positive outlook and an infinitely more successful career. I spent all of my newfound money on travelling. I made loads of new friends. I (eventually) stopped dating emotionally unavailable knobheads. I even learned how to dance in public sober.

Catherine Gray

Every addiction story wants a villain. But America has never been able to decide whether that villain is the substance or the user. Removing alcohol was one of the best decisions I have made in my adult life. I was thinking about booze all the time. Somebody once asked me how I define sobriety, and my response was 'liberation from dependence.' It seems there are two kinds of American writers. Those who drink, and those who used to.

Leslie Jamison

I figured out early on that the most important parts of life, for me, would be sobriety, relationships, love, and faith. The thing that I tried to do for so long is numb out the brutal. That's what addiction is — it's a hiding place from pain and numbing out. If you numb the brutal, you don't get to experience the beautiful. The first bit of sobriety will be hell. Then—after a long while—it will be slices of heaven every single day. You can do hard things, like wait out hell to get to heaven.

Glennon Doyle

As a Muslim, he would not drink alcohol, which is forbidden. That's why I don't drink alcohol. I don't party. Just trying to be a good follower.

Enes Kanter Freedom

I drank very heavily in my 20s and 30s. It's what we did. I was a musician. I quit drinking alcohol in my 30s, and I did a lot of things differently than I hadn't done before, because I wanted to not have the future that I saw coming. I don't know how to drink alcohol in a normal way. If you have any indication of problem drinking in your life, get help now. If you have a history of drinking problems in your family, do not take chances: Keep that switch turned off. Although forgoing alcohol can be difficult, you'll never be sorry you made this decision.

Arthur Brooks

Gravy these past ten years. Alive, sober, working, loving and being loved by a good woman. I'm a recovered alcoholic. I'll always be an alcoholic, but I'm no longer a practicing alcoholic. For years I didn't do anything except try to stay sober. I made it my priority. I didn't care if I never wrote another thing, if only he could stay sober and alive. Don't weep for me… I'm a lucky man.

Raymond Carver

You see, even though back when I was drinking I thought nothing bad ever happened to me, something did. Time passed. A lot of time passed. In bars, at parties with people I didn't care for. It was always the drink. It wasn't about love or reading the Sunday paper in bed. Or housebreaking a puppy. Or anything that people call 'life.' It was about drinking. So actually, something bad, very bad, did happen to me. I wasted my life. And now, what little I have left, I want. And If I was going to be completely sober for the rest of my life… then the life I lived needed to be a life from which I did not seek escape. Now I am absolutely happy in my life. I'm pretty happy, and I've certainly accomplished a lot, and I accomplished everything because I don't drink. That's the only variable. Nothing else in my life changed except I stopped drinking. But I had no idea how to fill the day when I got sober.

Augusten Burroughs

I have never missed drinking. No, I've missed drinking five or six times in the 23 years I've been sober. In my experience, sobriety makes good on the sparkle that booze/drugs/numbing promises but never delivers. I stopped drinking and smoking and went to my first Alcoholics Anonymous meeting on May 12, 1996. The not drinking is the easy part. The working the program, doing these fearless inventories of who I am and how I tap out of pain… that was the real work.

Brené Brown

I came out of it all knowing there was a better version of Steve Sarkisian inside of me. I wanted it for myself, but I wanted it for the people who love me and care about me. I'm proud of the work that I've done. But I will say when you battle what I battle, you have to work on it every day. How do I be the best version of Steve Sarkisian today?

Then tomorrow, hopefully, I'm better tomorrow. And then so on and so forth. I'm not going to focus on [the past]. I'm going to focus on today. I feel good in knowing the things that I'm doing, whether personally or professionally, are what are best for Steve Sarkisian.

Steve Sarkisian

There is a place for alcohol in life, but the effects of sobriety are strong, especially elective sobriety, which is choosing to be sober without needing to be – and feeling the strength that comes from that. The benefits of elective sobriety are so strong, it's really, really easy for you to just never want to reintroduce it.

Naval Ravikant

I wouldn't be able to have the life that I have now had it not been for me getting sober. I've been sober for almost nine, for nine years now and everything really powerfully good in my life has happened in my sobriety. One thing I do wish is I had gotten sober sooner. Um I do feel like I wasn't aware that I could be a happy person sober. I'm so proud that our kids will never ever see me intoxicated. I'm so proud that I have built a life that feels not boring.

Abby Wambach

Sobriety can often be viewed as a finish line. Rather, living in recovery is a choice that requires you to recommit day after day after day. Staying sober for me is one day at a time, sometimes one moment at a time. I had to rebuild my life from stocking shelves at a grocery store and going to meetings every day. But I felt better about my life at 11 months sober than I ever had playing in the NFL.

Darren Waller

Living sober is a great feeling. Being in the moment is important—how you react, respond, create. Now my mission is probably to help people who have the same problem... understand addiction and understand that it's a brain disease. I'm sober now, but it's an everyday struggle. I have an addiction. I'll always have an addiction. It never goes away. Any person that's an alcoholic or has any type of mental disease when it comes to drugs or alcohol... that's all an addict is, is mentally you're sick. I went to rehab and did some other things. I'm now feeling amazing. I'm alive, sober, and happy.

Lamar Odom

I am Muslim, I never drink. You want a better life? Start with better habits. Discipline every day, until discipline becomes you. Every man is addicted to something. Some smoke, some drink, some chase girls, some waste time. But a real man is addicted to discipline. Alcohol and girls stand in a way of an athlete. They make him weak. Discipline is the best addiction.

Khabib Nurmagomedov

I won't touch alcohol, religion is very important to me. I respect the rules of Islam and I pray five times a day, always. I have a chef who cooks for me, I like to eat healthy. I don't drink; I've never tried it in my life. I came to play football, not to drink alcohol.

Sadio Mané

What happens with fighters, we leave that ring that we've dedicated our lives to and all of a sudden you are burdened by drugs and alcohol and it becomes the thing. It can do one of two things: make you a better man by quitting, or it kills you. I learned that I had character defects, that I was allergic to alcohol and drugs, and that I had an obsession with all the bad stuff. But thank God that I woke and that I had good people around me to support me. There's not much more I can say about it. You have to want to be a better person.

Sugar Ray Leonard

Sex, bad character, drugs and alcohol are killing athletics. I'll actually enjoy my life by going to sleep, rather than going to a club. Only the disciplined ones are free in life. If you are undisciplined, you are a slave to your moods and your passions.

Eliud Kipchoge

I'm not someone who needs to go out drinking to enjoy myself. If I need to relax, I take my dogs out for a walk or I play a round of golf. I can't remember the last time I went to a club. I love just settling down and having a barbecue with friends at my house. It's not a monk's lifestyle, it's just all things in moderation.

Harry Kane

Today I celebrate 20 years of sobriety. What a journey it has been. Alcohol is a low vibrational substance that keeps you in emotional pain and suffering. My recovery must come first so that everything I love in life doesn't have to come last. Without my sobriety, I got nothing.

Theo Fleury

I started drinking when I was like 12 years old because I saw my dad drinking. When I became an adult, I started getting my own beer. The first time I tried it, I fell in love with it. I became addicted right away. Any time I would feel bad or feel good, that was like my scapegoat. The drinking started increasing as years started going on. And then it led to the drugs. I would medicate myself with the drugs and alcohol. People say, 'Don't do drugs, just drink.' Alcohol is a drug. And I know if I do one I'm going to do the other. From the numerous recovery attempts I've made, I've learned that alcohol inevitably leads back to the other substances. I got to a point in my life where I was just sick and tired of just basically being sick and tired. There were times I would literally be crying going to a liquor store.

Doc Gooden

It's discipline. You've just got to look at the bigger picture. All along I've tried not to get in that habit of drinking, because you don't need it if you want to keep performing at the highest level for a long time. I think you get more out of yourself if you don't drink. I don't think I'll really ever drink. I don't think I'll want to. My dad used to drink a lot so that's one of the reasons why I don't. My mum has said over the years 'try not to drink if you can'.

Jermain Defoe

Today when I look back, it's like I was another person. I wouldn't wish it on my worst enemy, to be in the grip of it. It's hell. You could call it a coping mechanism, but that would be an excuse. I just drank too much. Getting sober was one of the three pivotal events in my life, along with becoming an actor and having a child. Of the three, finding sobriety was the hardest thing. My own life, my personal life, is immeasurably better from just not living in a fog. I'm in a really good place now because I quit drinking. A lot of that is down to my sobriety. I can't be my authentic self without sobriety. That and my spiritual life are the only things that can't be taken from me.

Gary Oldman

I don't drink as I would rather do normal things with my friends and family. It's not the fact that I choose not to drink alcohol. I just don't like the taste of it. Playing computer games or watching a DVD is my idea of relaxing rather than going to nightclubs or that kind of thing. I don't drink and I don't go to nightclubs — that's why I'm so quick.

Gareth Bale

Partying was, I felt, a defining feature of my personality, and sobriety was really lonely at the beginning. It is an act of rebellion to remain present, to go against society's desire for you to numb yourself, to look away. But we must not look away. Sobriety has given me a level of creative freedom. Now, I can move through the world with so much more freedom and independence. I'm so much more in tune with what I want, what I like and what I want to make.

Florence Welch

I just had 19 years sober. There is an absolute change, and it took me about a year before I was comfortable playing consistently and sober. But I kept at it and I'm always so grateful. When you get sober, it's like you've been given your life back. You can actually see and feel things again. It's a whole new world. Alcohol was the one thing that was destroying my life. It was all about the next drink, the next fix. It was all just chaos and destruction.

Slash

When I finally got sober I had this moment of clarity. I got a message, a little thought that said, do you want to live or die? And I said I want to live. And suddenly the relief came and my life has been amazing. I am not infallible, and that is a very crucial fact I hope people understand. I'm sober and I'm happy being sober. I like it and I like who I am. I reflect on how sobriety – and the willingness to confront my past – has completely transformed my life. Over the past 24 years of sobriety, I've experienced profound joy, but not without significant challenges.

Nikki Sixx

I was always a drinker but I didn't know I was an alcoholic. None of my friends thought I was an alcoholic, and neither did I. I'd look at other people and think, 'They look fine and happy… how do they do it? They seem to be enjoying this ride called life.' Now I get to feel that way too. I know that I could drink if I wanted to, but I choose not to. If you're newly sober, keep at it, it gets so so awesome.

Sia

No more hangovers, no more chaos, just getting on with life. I don't see myself as a former alcoholic. I'm just Rob who doesn't drink. I just don't even think about drinking anymore. I haven't had a drink for 19 years. I just don't even think about drinking anymore.

Robbie Williams

My life has changed dramatically since I got sober. I used to be a very violent person when I drank. Sobriety has given me everything back that alcohol took away. I found God and I stopped drinking. I don't need the crutch of alcohol to have fun or be creative. Every day is a new challenge, but I wouldn't trade my sober life for anything.

Dave Mustaine

Sobriety is not a daily struggle, but it's a daily effort. I have to be proactive about my recovery. I think going to rehab was the best decision that I've ever made. I choose happiness over depression, I choose fulfillment over trying to fill an empty void. I have purpose now. Those are all things that drugs and alcohol strip away from me immediately.

Macklemore

I've been sober since my early twenties. I just felt like I was chasing chaos and making my life difficult, all the time thinking I was having fun. I didn't think it was very good for my life, and I immediately felt a change when I quit drinking. It feels very nice to not be putting myself in danger, to be waking up in the mornings and not thinking, 'Oh my god, who am I going to hear from? What did I do?' It's a life lived without dread and fear and it's lovely.

Christina Ricci

Every time I'd go out drinking I was looking for something new. But it was the same every time. I'd wake up in some bed with some person, I had a hangover and a show to do. And the truth is, it was the same every time. But now life is... pretty interesting without the alcohol.

James Hetfield

I don't drink. I used to drink, then I drank too much, and I had to stop. When you stop drinking, you lose some things — but you gain a lot more. You get new kinds of connections and new things that matter. In your 40s, you just stop pretending. You fill your life with work and family and people you love. There's no time for inauthenticity — and honestly, that makes everything a lot easier.

John Mulaney

I'm happier now than I've ever been. Sobriety didn't take anything from me – it gave me back. Am I an alcoholic? I may not be. I don't know. But I also know that in the situation I'm in, with temptations what they are, I have no room for alcohol in my life. I don't know how to do it like a gentleman. I don't know how to have one drink.

Shia LaBeouf

Six months of not drinking and getting fit isn't the cure all you think it's going to be. The rogue waves still come, and that's when your character is built. At first I was completely sober from both alcohol and weed, and then when I started using weed again I felt like I wasn't sober anymore. Sometimes I get high because I don't want to feel my feelings... I used to do that with alcohol.

Chelsea Handler

I can't tell you how much better my life is without that shit. My clarity and dynamics and directness with my friends, with my physical self and endeavors, with my creative process in the studio and live. I don't miss anything about the way I used to be, because I'm too satisfied with how I feel without it. I do miss certain components, but it's completely outbalanced by the benefits. I had some great times, but those great times don't measure up to the times that I'm having now, sober. Alcohol-induced great times are a bit fleeting, where sober great times have a stronger sense of permanence to them, for me. The memories are clearer, they're more sincere.

Ben Harper

My whole life has changed. What sobriety has taught me is to take things as they come and enjoy every moment of every day. I have big dreams, big aspirations, but where my life is at now is just trying to be as present as possible. My life feels so good now that I wouldn't give that up for anything. There is freedom in sobriety, and I am a living example of that. I am deeply grateful every day.

Lucy Hale

It was a matter of surrendering to sobriety. I was sober for a couple of weeks and after that I knew that I would never go back. I know I can only speak for one day at a time. I know I'm not going to drink today. And I gained so much by giving it up. I regained my life. Let the demons chase me and they can knock all they want. I'm not home.

John Goodman

I finally found the courage to ask for help and I am now 10 years sober. Sobriety has allowed me to live a life beyond my wildest dreams.

David Furnish

I lived with my alcoholic father from then until I was 16. Those who don't devise a positive way to feel significant may end up taking drastic measures to make themselves feel good, like turning to alcohol or engaging in frequent arguments. When you're living in a beautiful state, you don't need drugs or alcohol to enjoy your life.

Tony Robbins

Your life definitely changes. You pick up other things, you know, but nothing as detrimental as drinking. All it took was one book for me to quit drinking. I was still drinking at the time and I wasn't ready to give up drinking, but I knew at some point I would probably have to, so I bought the same Allen Carr book, his method for drinking. I had a really bad hangover in Cleveland in 2011 and I flew home and I read the book and then I was done drinking and it worked like that quickly. Once I stopped drinking, I realized I never want to go back.

Nikki Glaser

My life is very quiet, and I like it that way... there's a level of contentment that I experience now that is so much more rewarding than the highs and lows I used to have when I was drinking. You can drink all the green juice, dodge all the gluten, and run around town in all the fancy yoga pants you like—but it means nothing if you're not also addressing your mental, emotional, and spiritual well-being.

Ruby Warrington

Alcohol is small and irrelevant in my life. I am thankful that I never have to drink again!. I was drinking more than two bottles of wine a night. It wasn't that there was always a reason to drink. It was just that there was never a reason not to. If you could sum up my relationship with alcohol in a single word that word would be freedom. I drink as much as I want whenever I want to, I just haven't wanted to have a drink in five years now.

Annie Grace

I really love being sober. Alcohol doesn't fit into my life. I hate losing a day to something so dumb. It just is so incredibly... it's so unproductive. It's like the opposite of everything I love, which is like accomplishments and doing things and self-improvement. If you care about getting things done, drinking is the enemy.

Casey Neistat

I just felt like I was chasing chaos and making my life difficult, all the time thinking I was having fun. So it feels very nice to not be putting myself in danger, to be waking up in the mornings and not thinking, 'Oh my god, who am I going to hear from? What did I do?' The difference between not drinking and drinking for me is a happier life. It's much better. I don't miss drinking. Getting sober gave me joy, happiness and peace.

Ewan McGregor

Sobriety has given me everything I've ever wanted. I gave up on smoking, drinking and doing drugs years ago. My new addiction is running. I run three miles every day. I've been sober since the accident, but I've replaced all of my bad addictions with good ones.

Travis Barker

After you start the first steps, and you start working your way towards being a more functional person, and a sober person, a clear-headed person, you start seeing the results. I can't really have anything stronger than a Tylenol. It's been about six and a half years since I've had anything like a controlled substance or any alcohol. I'm now just a much more joyful, aware person than I was then. I'm more confident, and I don't have so many things to be ashamed of or afraid of. And I'm surrounded by people who I genuinely feel care about me. Plus, you know, I can go for a walk with my wife and not be sweaty and out of breath after 15 minutes, so that's nice, too. So now I look back on it with nothing but fond memories, and I see it as sort of this beautiful renaissance in my life that made everything that's happened possible.

Jason Isbell

Most of my buddies are dead. And for some reason, I am not. I was the guy that people pointed at and said, 'If I ever get like that, I'm going to quit.' And here I am, 30 plus years sober, telling you it's possible. It wasn't like you flick a switch, and you're sober. It takes a while. You have to learn how to do everything all over again. I learned how to take care of myself and then play in front of people. My life has got better beyond my wildest imagination.

Joe Walsh

I have no use for alcohol. I never had a drink in my life.

Jackie Robinson

There was a period of adjustment. There was a time, three or four years in, where I thought I had lost my mojo. I had lived my life with reckless abandon to great effect—just pushing every boundary that was in front of me. If there was a fence, I'm gonna step over it. And then to be in this thing where if you jump over the fence, you wake up in a blue suit. In a cell. It kind of turned me into a cautious person. I was really nervous and scared about everything for a while. I would drive the car at 49 miles an hour, with nothing in the car, and still think I was going to get pulled over and yanked out of my life by some authority figure. Sober people around me kept reminding me "More will be revealed" and "Just keep going," "Don't quit till the miracle happens," and all those sayings they have. And lo and behold, they were right. I thought my mojo was gone, but you find a new kind of mojo. The important thing is to know that there is a way out. And the life at the other end of that is a beautiful life.

Trey Anastasio

I had to learn a different way to be in the world without drugs and alcohol. What 'high' means to me now is my family, my friends, this rollercoaster musical journey I'm on. Playing live is where I always feel high. I chose sobriety 19 years ago and I'm never looking back.

Keith Urban

People think I'm a punk, and wild, and out of control but I'm really healthy. I'm vegan, I'm a straight-edge, and I like being home alone. I don't drink at all. I don't need that to be happy. I'm just not really around it. I just naturally don't gravitate towards it. Because I think there's something that most people find quite charismatic about people that are like carefree and live that way, but I see so past that. I'm like, "I'm really sorry that you're in pain, and I'm really sorry that you need a crutch, and I'm really sorry that this is your way to tune out from the world."

Soko

Sobriety, for me, has been more than abstaining from substances – it's learning to take care of myself in a way I never did before. In sobriety, one looks for a balance and equilibrium. As I'd become famous, there was always a bottle of champagne backstage, and, as my workload increased, I had been smoking more and more weed, until I was smoking first thing in the morning. And when you're stoned, it's harder to keep a balance. Sobriety is a real, real gift. You honor that gift by shining, by showing up as the best version of yourself.

RuPaul

I wrote a song called "Sober", which is actually really dark. I was at a party at my own house, I didn't want to be there, I didn't want anyone else there. And I had this line in my head saying, 'How do I feel this good sober?', it's not just about alcohol, it's about vices, we all have different ones. We try to get away from ourselves, and find our 'true selves' and then we do these things that take us so far from the truth, I guess that 'Sober' is 'How do I feel this good when it's just me, without anything to lean on?'

Pink

I'm grateful to be alive, that's for sure. And that gives me the possibility to do anything. Everything starts with sobriety. Because if you don't have sobriety, you're going to lose everything that you put in front of it, so my sobriety is right up there. I'm an extremely grateful guy.

Matthew Perry

Looking back at my wild drinking days, I really never imagined that I would be excited about being sober. When you are on the other side of things, you have such a profoundly different perspective on life. On this side, you realize it's something to be celebrated. Personally, being sober means that I operate better and I function better; I believe I am meant to be that way. Although I'm just returning to where I'm supposed to be, it remains important to me. I live a very simple life and that is very appealing to me. My time is spent focused on practicing and mastering the things I am passionate about as an artist and as a person.

Kat Von D

I don't discuss this a lot. I discuss it every now and then when it makes sense. I'm 39 years sober. I got sober when I was just about to turn 27. I'm glad I got sober when I did, because not many people get sober when they're young.

Alec Baldwin

If you would have told me 365 days ago that I would be sober, happy, and about to be a mumma I would have laughed in your face. Life is truly amazing when you do the work. If you are new to sobriety stick to it life really does get good. I can wholeheartedly confess that I'm finally at peace with myself and truly starting to understand what true happiness is.

Kelly Osbourne

The power that my addiction had over me… I never thought that I could stop. It became my identity. I didn't know who I was without it. I really started to reflect and see like, 'Okay, I'm not okay." I was not happy. I was not at peace. I needed to better my life. That's not the lifestyle that I want to live. September 14th will be my three years of sobriety… three years of happiness, three years of peace, three years of love, kindness, forgiveness, everything. This is not a one and done situation. This is a lifestyle for me. I'm not going back.

Blac Chyna

We decided to do Dry January. Those months without alcohol showed me how much better I feel. Dry January was our reset. It has been a wake up call about how much we were drinking. We spent 2,869 dollars on alcohol in December. We were binge drinking. It was an absurd number of drinks. I'm now drinking less than I have in years. I've basically stopped and felt much better in many ways.

Amy Robach

I like to have clean-living people around me. I like a clean band. I don't like drugs. I don't like alcohol. I'm not one of those people who stays up until four in the morning eating pizza and drinking beer. If I wasn't focusing on my family I was focusing on music. I took music very seriously. It was my outlet, it was my drug. All my teenage years in bars, I never took a drink. I certainly could've gone off track many, many times in my youth. Just wasn't interested.

Shania Twain

I don't do clubs. I don't drink. I don't smoke. I've never had a drink in my life. I'm sober. I've never been interested. Nobody ever believes it. I'm 31 and I've never, ever, ever had a drink or done a drug in my entire life. I stick with Diet Coke and Crystal Light and water.

Jennifer Hudson

Wine took over because I knew it looked better and was linked to some health benefits. I found myself drinking two bottles of wine on the couch. Once I was going for that third bottle of wine, I said, 'you've got a problem,' and it was cold turkey that day. I just stopped. I've been sober for over 20 years. The journey to self-love can be a brutal process. Especially in those moments when we must deny ourselves that which is familiar but harmful. My sobriety comes before everything because without it I have nothing.

Jada Pinkett Smith

I don't do much partying now. I'm a very serious guy. I'm a professional, so I've stopped drinking. It was clearly affecting what I do. I was annoyed I hadn't been getting enough done, hangovers were taking over. Things are a bit less fun without drinking alcohol, but my live shows are a million times better now. I've had the best year of my life not drinking. It's been great.

Calvin Harris

Alcohol is probably the worst one to deal with. It's everywhere, so many people do it, it's socially acceptable and legal. I have made many mistakes in my life but each day is a chance to start again. Atone for mistakes and grow. For anyone who wakes up thinking 'oh god not again' I promise you there's a way. My life since getting sober is so much greater than it ever would be.

Jamie Campbell Bower

It is most emphatically true that the chance for leading a happy and prosperous life is immensely improved if only the man is decent, sober, industrious, and exercises foresight and judgment. I have never been drunk or in the slightest degree under the influence of liquor.

Theodore Roosevelt

Building new habits is hard enough as it is, and I'd made it even harder by being hungover once or twice every couple of weeks. There is no chance that I'm going to do morning meditation or reading when I'm desperately holding on for dear life in the midst of a hangover, let alone if I'm still asleep. By having more stability in my schedule, I was able to build the consistency that I needed to embed these habits. In fact, I built a meditation habit five years ago—the first time I ever went sober—and I still use it today.

Chris Williamson

I stopped drinking in 2003 because I felt I couldn't be fully present in my life. Everybody has their own journey and I'm not interested in telling other people what to do but I know that this was a decision that I've never regretted. After 21 years sober, I don't even think about drinking. I think about living and thriving. There's nothing I could drink to improve the way I'm feeling right now.

Elle MacPherson

I didn't realize what I was falling into when it came to drinking. I really— it became habit, it became a routine, it was something that was very easy to do and a part of the daily routine.

Joe Namath

When I gave up dope and alcohol, my immediate feeling was 'I've saved my life, but there'll be a price because I'll have nothing that buzzes me anymore.' But I enjoyed my kids. My wife loved me and I loved her... And I discovered that the writing was enough. Stupid thing is that probably it always had been. Only a lunatic—a masochistic lunatic—would make booze a regular part of his life.

Stephen King

Today marks three years—zero booze in my life. And man I'll just say for anybody that's wanting to take the leap or thinking about doing it, I hope you do because every aspect of my life—my family life, my personal life, my business career, everything—has been net positive.

Shawn Ryan

Why, I never drank a drop of liquor in my life. I have never tasted liquor in my life. I have no liquors in my house... I shall provide cold water— nothing else. Let us make it as unfashionable to withhold our names from the temperance pledge.

Abraham Lincoln

I stayed away from drinking and drugs in high school and only experimented a bit in college. These days I don't really drink at all; it's just something I chose to step away from as an adult. I don't condemn people who do; I've just never wanted to. I don't do things that are dangerous to myself. I don't want to hurt myself. I'm one of those people who just doesn't get much out of alcohol, so it was easy for me to give it up.

Natalie Portman

My sobriety has been the key to freedom—the freedom to be me, to not be looking in the mirror in the reflection and trying to see somebody else. I look in the mirror. I see myself. I accept myself. And I move on because you know what? The world is filled with things we need to do.

Jamie Lee Curtis

By my mid-twenties I realized it was either the serious writing or the drinking, and I chose to let the drinking go. When the medication causes the disease, a positive feedback loop has been established. The goal isn't just to stop the habit, it's to become the person who wouldn't pick it up again. You need an adventure. You need to get out there and have something to do. That's the substitute for the addiction.

Jordan Peterson

I resolved to prioritize my recovery above everything else and cleared my schedule completely for a year. I genuinely believe I would not have maintained my sobriety had I not devoted that entire year to my recovery program.

Elton John

I can abuse alcohol if the demons get me. I'll go on a bender. I was drinking too much. So I said, "This time I'm going to stick it through for a month. It was one of the best things I ever did.

Billy Joel

I wasn't ready to get sober. I was sneaking it on planes, sneaking it in bathrooms, sneaking it throughout the night. Nobody knew. I no longer support my 'California sober' ways. Sober sober is the only way to be.

Demi Lovato

It was not like I had this huge bottom moment; it was really just this moment of 'Why am I doing this? I started having panic attacks with drinking... when I would feel hung over, it would be until 7:00 p.m. the next day. I did 'sober January' and just decided to keep going. It honestly just started out as I was just going to do sober January, and then turned into almost five years. I wanted to share this because I am really proud of myself. Yesterday I celebrated 6 Months of Sobriety. It's not something I planned on but after the long journey of getting here I can honestly say I have never been more proud of myself in my entire life.

Rumer Willis

It is now 10 years since I used drugs or drank alcohol and my life has improved immeasurably. Whatever I endure in recovery, I need never again suffer the indignity of active addiction, the despair and hopelessness.

Russell Brand

You want your life to be different? Do something different. Small changes create big shifts. Go to bed early. Stop drinking for a week. Understanding alcohol is understanding that it often borrows happiness from tomorrow.

Jay Shetty

I don't drink alcohol. It's poison for your body. If you want to be the best, you have to sacrifice. Training is vital, but living a calm life is just as important so you can be at your best physically and mentally; I spend my free time with family and friends to stay relaxed and positive.

Cristiano Ronaldo

I had this ideal idea of wine tastings and all that — which is what it was at first. And that's a very subtle thing. I mean, I drank the best. I kept it to two bottles, and I would drink them both over the course of the day. I've done a lot of damage to the body. I've been clean, ten years this December. I stopped at 60, and I haven't had a thimble's worth since. Things are opening up for me now.

Denzel Washington

I gave up drinking alcohol. The time between 1998 and 2005 was especially bad. During that time I avoided looking in the mirror, because I didn't like the person who was looking back at me. I don't miss that partying life; everything is better without the chaos of alcohol and drugs. Not drinking makes me a lot happier. I want to lead a calm life.

Naomi Campbell

I haven't had alcohol in years, and I don't miss it at all. My body is my vehicle; if I expect a lot from it, I have to treat it with love, not alcohol. Before I was surviving; now, with healthier choices, I'm really living. Sobriety helps me stop running away from myself and actually live my life.

Gisele Bündchen

I don't drink. I've never tried a drug... it's not like I decided on these strict lifestyle choices and I'm enforcing them. It's just something that I genuinely don't have a desire for. Drinking isn't my thing.

Blake Lively

I one hundred percent know I like me better sober. I one hundred percent know I get more done, I absolutely feel better in my body without it. And I am one hundred percent pissed that I can't be normal and have a cocktail with my husband on vacay without it turning into 8 and feeling like shit.

Chrissy Teigen

My addictions were very secret, very locked up; they shocked the people around me. Before getting sober, I would look in the mirror, call myself names, and completely despise myself. I feel like an entirely different person now that I'm sober. I learned that the saying 'a leopard doesn't change its spots' is wrong; the idea that I could truly change kept me going. Sobriety is a wonderful way to live; it saved me.

I have a child and my relationship is brilliant I'm a very, very happy, content, sober man.

Kit Harington

I said no drinks, no sex, all the big things... But still, it's just one of those things I haven't done, and I don't see any benefit to doing it. You're always reading about people getting DUIs. So many bad things that happen and wind up in the paper are alcohol related, so by not drinking, it saves me, my team and my family a lot of trouble.

Tim Tebow

8. Quotes on the Spiritual Side

God, Peace, Higher Power, Inner Life

My addiction wasn't about alcohol—it was about the collapse of my inner life. You don't think your way out of addiction. You live your way into a spiritual solution. Alcohol robbed me of my integrity. Recovery gave me my soul back. Staying sober requires a daily spiritual practice—however you define that. Spirituality is important because it is reality. And we are not human beings having a spiritual experience. We are spiritual beings having a human experience.

Rich Roll

I pray every day—I roll out of bed and get on my knees before I do anything else: 'God, keep the desire to drink and drug from me this day.' That's all I need to say about that.

Samuel L. Jackson

I meditate and then I do my vocal warm up and then I go in the bathroom and I always kind of kneel down in front of the toilet. And there's a reason that I do that. Because I used to drink too much and it put me in front of that toilet and I like to remind myself how grateful I am that today I haven't had to do that. Phish shows are completely wrapped up into my spiritual life at this point. Especially since becoming sober almost 12 years ago. It's taken years — and it will probably be a lifetime — of unraveling how far I had strayed from my inner compass. I'm so grateful that it didn't kill me. It could have.

Trey Anastasio

I was in a washroom in my house, and I knew that eventually I was going to die. I just basically said, please, God, take away the obsession to drink and do drugs. Next thing I know, 30 minutes goes by and I went, holy cow, I said my prayers have been answered. That was Sept.

18, 2005, and I haven't had a drink or a drug since that day. Today I celebrate 20 years of sobriety. What a journey it has been.

Theo Fleury

I tried so many times to get sober on my own for eight years in a row. I'd get three years and three months and I'd go back to drinking. I'd get a year in recovery, or being sober, and I'd go back to drinking. I would try to stop drinking, and I couldn't. There was a two-decade struggle. I never reached out for help, or hardly, because of the stigma of addiction. Most people did not know anything about my struggle. But there was a point in time where I guess I was suicidal at the end of my drinking. And there was a point in time where I just, I had faith that there is God, but I wasn't part of an organized religion. And I was out walking. I always get emotional when I tell this story, but I just said, "If there's anybody out there, I need help." And I've been sober since I uttered those words. So, you know, that was a miracle for me, because I spent a lot of years relapsing. And I'm so grateful to be here today.

Kathryn Burgum

Before, I was at war with myself and I didn't want to admit it. The beginning of sobriety was brutal. There was nothing pretty about it. No confidence. No peace. Just survival, one minute at a time. I just prayed, "Heavenly Father, give me the strength to overcome addiction and the challenges that come with it." I am now sober and grateful.

Oksana Baiul

When I drank, I knelt on the bathroom floor to throw up. When I got sober, I did it to pray. I got down on my knees to pray even though I wasn't sure what I was praying to, only what I was praying for: don't drink, don't drink, don't drink. The second time I got sober, I started praying with a sense of purpose. It felt good to kneel on the bathroom floor for different reasons than I'd knelt on them before.

Leslie Jamison

Sobriety to me is a magical. It's a path that leads me deeper and deeper to the truth of things, to the truth of my heart, to what I would call God, what some people would just call love or truth. Sobriety to me is not just not drinking. Or not doing something, right? It's a discipline. It's a religion to me really, if a religion is just a set of ideas that gets us further to the truth of things. By the grace of God and the program of AA, I have been sober for many years now. I got sober when I was twenty-five. I figured out early on that the most important parts of life, for me, would be sobriety, relationships, love, and faith.

Glennon Doyle

Talking about spiritual activity to a secular audience is like doing card tricks on the radio. I thought faith was a feeling. My intellect told me this was insane. The only way I was able to do it was through practice. I'd been trying to get sober and not really listening to the ways you're supposed to do it, and somebody said, 'pray on your knees every day for 30 days and see if you stay sober.' What keeps you sober is love and connection to something bigger than yourself.

Mary Karr

I used to bargain with God at the toilet after drinking too much, promising I would quit if the suffering stopped, and then I would go right back to it. I come from a line of alcoholics—my grandfather, my father, and I all had that vulnerability—so I had every reason to take alcohol seriously. The strongest 'treatment' for alcoholism is a deep, life reorienting religious conversion.

Jordan Peterson

People often think football saved my life. Really, recovery and my relationship with God saved my life. Today marks 7 years of continuous sobriety from drugs and alcohol by the grace of God! It's really just been a moment-by-moment process of trying to seek God despite my ego, foster connection despite my desire to isolate, and look for what I can give to a situation rather than what I can get out of it.

Darren Waller

I got better for one reason: I surrendered. I prayed to be spared another day of guilt and depression and addiction. I couldn't continue, and I couldn't stop, either. It was a horrible downward spiral that I had to pull out of or die. So how am I here? I can only shrug and say, 'It's a God thing.' It's the only possible explanation. Alone, I couldn't win this battle. With Jesus, I couldn't lose. I now go to sleep every night with a clear mind and a clear conscience

Josh Hamilton

At that point I knew I couldn't do it on my own. I got on my knees and, for the first time in my life, I knew I couldn't stop going to the pub on my own. I was crying. When I arose, I was bouncing with excitement. I had faith that everything was going to be alright.

Tyson Fury

I knew I had come to a crossroads in my life. With the grace of God, I got sober and I saved my life. I was a new man, a renewed man. I proudly have not had a drink since 1998. I feel like a different person now that I'm sober. I feel much better now that I don't drink and have straightened my life out. I wouldn't trade these 12 years for nothing. I'm at peace.

Brett Favre

I got to 90 days being clean and sober by putting God first, admitting to Him that I had a problem using, and taking it one day at a time. I remember when I got like 90 days sober I was just like, holy man, like it was like the first time I'd ever done something for myself.

Theo Von

I stopped drinking. It was will power. It was prayer. It was really hard. I didn't want to go to rehab. I believe that anything man can do for me, God can do for me in a greater way. It's just a decision and something I'm not doing right now.

Mary J Blige

I think that faith and sobriety coincided for me because of how I saw the principles of faith performed. And as far as the very person I was, I don't miss that person at all. That person was very selfish and hurt a lot of people. I'm able to say that I like myself so much more now.

Julien Baker

My identity shifted when I got into recovery. From that day until this, I have never failed to pray in the morning, on my knees, asking for help, and at night to express gratitude for my life and, most of all, for my sobriety. I choose to kneel because I feel I need to humble myself when I pray, and with my ego, this is the most I can do. The compulsion was taken away at that moment, and as far as I was concerned, that was physical evidence that my prayers had been answered. In all the time I've been sober, I have never once seriously thought of taking a drink or a drug.

Eric Clapton

The complete transformation of consciousness that is possible through the miraculous spiritual technology of the 12 Steps. You have to understand that I had tried quite literally everything the world had to offer to make myself feel better, to stop acting out, and to be emotionally healthy—from tons of therapy, to pharmaceuticals, to gurus of all manner, to plant medicine, to every kind of self-help and self-improvement pursuit out there—but nothing ever worked for me (meaning: nothing transformed my behavior) until I came into the rooms of 12-step and started really working those steps with an experienced, older, and very disciplined sponsor. All addicts operate from a place of infinite need that they're trying to fill with whatever finite source they're using, whether it's drugs, or alcohol, or cigarettes, or food, or shopping, or gambling, or gaming, or workaholism. Whatever the thing is that you're pouring into what we call the God-sized hole, it doesn't work.

Elizabeth Gilbert

I wasn't really actively pursuing any belief system. I was just sad. I was drinking and I was trying to find answers in the wrong places, and it wasn't until I got sober, which is — it's 17 years ago in July — that I really opened up my eyes to wanting to fix myself. I've been sober for a long time, but I don't feel like I was free from all of it until I found God.

Kat Von D

Sometimes you need a cold bucket of water in the face to sort of snap to, because you're dealing with a sort of malady of the soul, an obsession of the mind and a physical allergy. They call it the spiritual path for the psychopath. They say there's only three options: you go insane, you die or you quit. That's the harsh reality. The moment I reached for something greater than myself, everything changed. That's a miracle. For me, it is. Life didn't suddenly get perfect after I quit drinking—but it got real. The work, the peace, the relationships— they don't come easy, but they're real. For many, it is. If you're suffering from a spiritual malady, the cure is spiritual too.

Mel Gibson

I needed an excuse to drink and not feel the pain of everyday life and trauma. My toxic relationship with alcohol left me stagnant with closed eyes, hindering my growth and my healing. Hindering my ability to overcome fear. I'm letting go and letting God!

Ari Lennox

I've made a promise with God to never drink again. I had my conversation with God. I can't lie to Him. I said, 'I ain't doin' it no more, I ain't doin' it.' I see how the people around me appreciate it, I love it.

Allen Iverson

Forty-five years ago today, I had a wakeup call. I was heading for disaster, drinking myself to death. I got a message, a little thought, that said, 'Do you want to live or die?' I said, 'I want to live.' Some deep powerful thought or voice spoke to me from inside and said: 'It's all over. Now you can start living.' And suddenly the relief came, and my life has been amazing.

Anthony Hopkins

Three years sober today. September 14th will be my three years of sobriety… three years of happiness, three years of peace, three years of love, kindness, forgiveness, everything. Thank you God and the mercy of Jesus Christ for walking with me on this journey of healing and everlasting life. If you're struggling with sobriety, I promise you're not alone.

Blac Chyna

When I started, I took it one day at a time. Ultimately, I found that spirituality worked for me. I do think a spiritual and transcendent change is required for people to be free from addiction. When you start to drink, wank, eat, spend, obsess excessively you have lost your connection to the great power within you... it is your spirit calling and it craves connection. I need spirituality. I need God, or I cannot cope in this world

Russell Brand

I stopped drinking and I started going back to church. Drinking beer is easy. Trashing your hotel room is easy. But being a Christian, that's a tough call. That's real rebellion. I have absolutely no desire to ever put alcohol in my mouth again. You get addicted to being sober, that's all.

Alice Cooper

While I probably could have gone another ten years drinking, because that was my drug of choice, emotionally and spiritually I felt barren. I was drinking too much. It was like, I don't feel connected to myself. I don't feel connected to life. I don't feel connected to God, or spirit, or the universe. I don't feel connect to nature. That's a very painful place to be in. And I really wanted to find out why I felt disconnected, which is why I drank, because I felt disconnected. I stopped drinking because I felt I couldn't be fully present in my life, and it was a wonderful springboard of getting to know myself on a deeper level. I think that's the most important thing. You say I look incredible, but I feel that way. I just love that sense of vitality and I'm grateful for my life. I feel incredible.

Elle MacPherson

It is a disease of the soul and the mind, and it will tear up the people around you. It's a matter of hitting a personal bottom. I was tired of my excuses, I was tired of the shame and the guilt. So much energy to manage it. It was unmanageable. I said to whatever God that was watching over me: 'Help me! I will do what you want.' I'm a guy who doesn't like 'organized' anything but AA is just brilliant to me.

Tim Allen

I had to first admit to myself that my life was unmanageable, that a Higher Power could restore me to sanity, and that I was willing to turn my life over. People think the steps are about quitting drinking or getting sober. But the real purpose of the 12 Steps is changing yourself so everything else can change. I used to believe self-love is woo woo and for people out to lunch, but getting sober was my first act of self-love.

Kevin Kreider

I knew nothing about AA but they were incredibly helpful and welcoming. The meetings gave me a place to go and the support I needed for the first year and a half of my sobriety while I created a new life and developed other support systems.

Hayley Gibson

I finally quit drinking and doing drugs, and I walked into an AA meeting, and that was 12 years ago and I haven't looked back. Last week I marked 14 years clean, sober and smoke free.

Gregory Gourdet

I was never into drugs or alcohol. That was fortunate. I don't have a propensity to be addicted to those things. I have friends that are recovered alcoholics... their lives are so much better as a function of being sober. People who have alcohol use disorder, their main goal should be to quit alcohol completely. There are many pathways to recovery, and for a lot of people, AA and 12-step are incredibly helpful.

Andrew Huberman

I decided to stop drinking alcohol so that I could concentrate on my life and my relationship with God. My husband and I stopped taking alcohol to focus on our marriage and God.

Anerlisa Muigai

I just left an AA meeting. I have such a desire to want to keep this feeling and stay this way, and I'm willing to do whatever it takes. Being in recovery and leaving a place where you're in this little bubble and everything is safe around you, it's really hard. But there's nothing left in having a drink for me. I feel better not drinking. I feel whole again.

Lindsay Lohan

It only took me one more year to admit that I could no longer control my drinking. And finally, on July 7, 1986, I quit, and let a bunch of sober alcoholics teach me how to get sober, and stay sober. I do not at all understand the mystery of grace -- only that it meets us where we are but does not leave us where it found us.

Anne Lamott

I just really felt like alcohol wasn't serving me. I wanted to do whatever it took to make me feel better physically and spiritually.

Kyle Richards

Overcoming addiction was the biggest hurdle I've faced in my life. I physically, mentally, and chemically can't control my alcohol consumption once I take the first drink. God pulled me out of the pit so I could go back and pull more people out, and that's what I plan to do. My journey in sobriety is my badge of honor, not my shameful story.

Maxx Crosby

I went to Alcoholics Anonymous, went through the 12 steps and it changed me as a human being. The greatest thing that I ever did was to say 'I can't do this'... my ways got me here and it's not worked. So, I open myself up to something else. My life has been unbelievable since that day.

Tony Adams

I hit rock bottom and I started going to a 12-step program, and I've been sober ever since. There was a small voice in me that wanted to live... and I'm still sober now, so I am really grateful. I'd look at other people and think, 'They look fine and happy... how do they do it? They seem to be enjoying this ride called life.' Now I get to feel that way too.

Sia

People romanticize drinking, and even I romanticized it. But I can't be my authentic self without sobriety. That and my spiritual life are the only things that can't be taken from me.

Gary Oldman

Some of the higher vibrational feeling states that I used alcohol to attempt to access were relaxation, amusement, connection, pleasure, and transcendence. The good news is that I experience all these highs and more as a sober curious person. Alcohol is a weak imitation of the joy, inspiration, confidence, connection, and overall sense of aliveness that can only be generated from within. Could it be that joy was there all along, like a balloon held underwater always trying to bob to the surface?

Ruby Warrington

When I stopped drinking, I was that scared little kid again. And I managed to get some consecutive days of sobriety, and I went to some AA meetings, and I realized, "I can't say my life got better, but it stopped getting worse." And that was huge. So I stuck around. My life has got better beyond my wildest imagination. People often ask me if I believe in God, and I kinda have to, because I'm still here. I had not planned on living this long, and here I am.

Joe Walsh

Through the years of drinking and doing drugs, I always had this very specific voice inside of me that goes, 'One day you're gonna come to a crossroads… You're either gonna choose to get out of this shit or you're never gonna get out of it.' It has a lot to do with my dad and being born into a family with an alcoholic father. My job is to now maybe break that chain and do something different.

Keith Urban

I'm very grateful for being sober. I continue to partake in the 12-step program. I can be in Afghanistan, I can be in Japan, and go to a meeting and the room is full of alcoholics and people that did drugs like I did. Getting clean was the hardest — and best — thing I've ever done.

Steven Tyler

Somebody once asked me how I define sobriety, and my response was 'liberation from dependence'.

Leslie Jamison

The reward for total abstinence from alcohol seems, illogically enough, to be the capacity for becoming intoxicated without it.

Rebecca West

I don't drink anymore. I had to stop, because it wasn't fun – it was survival. I went to a 12-step meeting every day, sometimes twice a day. People talked about numbing the discomfort of being in their own skin, and then having to face themselves in the cold light of sobriety – that was my story too.

RuPaul

When I started, I took it one day at a time. Ultimately, I found that spirituality worked for me. I do think a spiritual and transcendent change is required for people to be free from addiction. Addicts and alcoholics have a spiritual craving and no language for it, so we anesthetize it.

Russell Brand

A decade ago I was super lost. Alcohol was pulling me further from myself, so I made the choice to stop drinking. It wasn't until I went teetotal that I was able to find myself. Ten years sober taught me that the life I wanted started when I quit drinking. It's been tough sometimes, but sobriety gave me clarity, confidence and peace. I'm grateful beyond words. I thought being sober meant my life would be over — it turned out to be the opposite.

Elsa Hosk

People want my story to be this after-school special where I just say, 'Oh look, I was an addict, and now I'm sober and that's it. And it's not as simple as that. It doesn't happen overnight. I realized that 12-step treatment was the best thing, and it was about not being ashamed of that. The community made a huge difference. The opposite of addiction is connection, and I really found that in 12-step.

Cara Delevingne

If anyone is out there and struggling in the first two years, it does get easier. It's given me a level of creative freedom. Now, I can move through the world with so much more freedom and independence. I'm so much more in tune with what I want, what I like and what I want to make. Sobriety is the best thing I ever did.

Florence Welch

I'm lucky to have found recovery through a 12-steps program almost 14 years ago and it's something that I still do regularly to this day. It gives me a lot of structure in my life. It's really the bedrock of my life and from it, all these wonderful things have been built. I'm less concerned with happy and I'm more into content. And I'm more than content.

Josh Peck

Alcohol silenced my intuition, blocked my dreams and chased my circulating fears of complacency. I haven't wanted or touched alcohol since October 2017 and it has been the best decision I've made for myself and for my family. I thought it was making me brave, I thought it was making me confident and it was actually the complete opposite. It was silencing me.

Jessica Simpson

Now I want to get through the rough night. And I found, in doing so, you just, you come out the other side with a more profound understanding of yourself and a gratefulness for those in your life. And for the birds and the trees and everything else.

Brad Pitt

Being in recovery has given me everything of value that I have in my life. Integrity, honesty, fearlessness, faith, a relationship with God, and most of all gratitude.

Rob Lowe

I was achieving everything I had dreamed of for 30 years. It all came to fruition, and I was the least happy I had ever been. I was closest to not wanting to live than I had ever been, despite having everything I had ever desired. I'm grateful for this realization because it made me understand that something much deeper was broken.

Dax Shepard

I'm in a lifestyle that I know is really working on a high road for my little journey, and there's so much peace finally being had where there were demons.

Drew Barrymore

When I got sober, I had no sense of self-worth and did not believe that I deserved better in life. I was complacent with my existence because I felt broken by my choices and thought that's what I deserved. Sobriety taught me I was wrong—every day I learn to forgive myself just a bit more.

Charlie Sheen

I wouldn't be here without sobriety. It gave me my life back — and everything good flows from that. I just started going [to Alcoholics Anonymous]. And I think it's changed my life. I'm much more comfortable in my own skin. Things are so much easier now. I'm in the best place that I've ever been in. I've never been this happy before.

Zac Efron

Trying to deal with fame, I got stupid and drank too much. Trying to find what it is to be a real human being and what it is to live through fame was hard. The loneliness of fame was messing with my head. But I feel fortunate that I've come out the other end.

Patrick Swayze

I was still going through a lot of crap, and I knew that I wanted to be on the road of intentionally finding my core happiness. I don't need anything to amplify my happiness. I feel high just on life. I recently went out to dinner with a friend, and I had ginger ale in a wine glass. And it felt like I was celebrating. Because for a long time, I leaned on it. Right now, I love how I feel more than how the alcohol makes me feel.

Valerie Bertinelli

I like life too much without it. Now that I'm completely free of it, I don't have any desire to ever drink again. I decided to quit drinking because I wanted to live my life, not blur my way through it. Sobriety gave me back my joy, my health, and my reason to wake up smiling.

Dick Van Dyke

Whoever I had become had to die. Whether I or anyone else accepted the concept of alcoholism as a disease didn't matter; what mattered was that when treated as a disease, those who suffered from it were most likely to recover.

Craig Ferguson

Alcohol was a buffer that made me disconnected from who I really was. I'm very serious about no alcohol, no drugs. Life is too beautiful.

Jim Carey

Drinking was destroying me, but that unused potential was a spiritual death It's the difference between existing and actually living. The typical question is, Is this bad enough for me to have to change? The question we should be asking is, Is this good enough for me to stay the same? And the real question underneath it all is, Am I free?

Laura McKowen

I never drank alcohol. I have a relative peace with myself. My faith gives me tranquility. By constant self-discipline and self-control you can develop greatness of character.

John Wooden

My secret nearly destroyed my life, but God's grace restored everything. By not telling people, it becomes more powerful. But when you put it out there in the open, just like I'm doing right now, it loses its power. Sobriety has given me everything that drugs and alcohol ever promised me.

Terry Crews

I dedicated myself to sobriety, and God told me that I would be rewarded and that he would show me just how good it can get. Where I am now, sobriety is serving me, and I'm creating from a different place – I have no outside influence besides me and my thoughts. It's like I'm experiencing a different type of high, a high on just life. I know that sounds so corny, but I'm serious!

Doechii

I don't drink, I don't smoke, I don't do drugs, I don't chase women, I don't do any of that stuff. I'm just trying to live a life that honors God and is a positive influence.

Tim Tebow

9. The Stars Who Quit Profiles

Alphabetical Order by first name / stage name. For their quotes on alcohol, reference *The Stars Who Quit Index* (pp 255 – 258)

50 Cent (Curtis Jackson) is a rapper, actor, and entrepreneur who broke through in 2003 when Get Rich or Die Tryin' sold about 872,000 copies in its first week, debuted at number one on the Billboard 200, and produced the number-one singles "In da Club" and "21 Questions" on the Billboard Hot 100. He released multi-platinum albums including The Massacre and sold over 30 million records worldwide. He won a Grammy Award and multiple Billboard Music Awards and American Music Awards. He expanded into business and television by founding G-Unit Records and G-Unit Film & Television and serving as executive producer of the STARZ series Power (2014–2020) and its spin-offs. His equity stake in Vitaminwater yielded an estimated $100 million payout when Coca-Cola acquired the brand in 2007.

Abby Wambach is a soccer player who scored 184 goals in 255 matches for the U.S. women's national team from 2001 to 2015, becoming international soccer's all-time leading scorer at the time of her retirement. She played in four FIFA Women's World Cups, winning the title in 2015, and earned Olympic gold medals in 2004 and 2012. She was named FIFA World Player of the Year in 2012. In professional leagues she won the 2003 Women's United Soccer Association championship and played across multiple U.S. leagues including WUSA, WPS, and NWSL. After retiring in 2015, she became an author and speaker, publishing the bestseller Wolfpack and expanding into leadership and organizational development through books, media, and public speaking.

Abraham Lincoln is a political leader who rose from Illinois state legislator and one-term U.S. congressman to national prominence through the 1858 Lincoln–Douglas debates on slavery's expansion. As the 16th president of the United States, elected in 1860 and reelected in 1864, he led the Union during the Civil War, issuing the Emancipation Proclamation in 1863 and supporting passage of the Thirteenth Amendment in 1865, which abolished slavery nationwide. His administration preserved the federal union after Confederate secession and oversaw wartime mobilization that expanded federal authority. He was assassinated in April 1865 shortly after the Confederacy's defeat, ending his presidency during the restoration..

Adele is a singer and songwriter whose debut album *19* (2008) reached number one on the UK Albums Chart and earned her the Grammy Award for Best New Artist in 2009. Her follow-up *21* (2011) topped the Billboard 200 for 24 weeks, produced the number-one singles "Rolling in the Deep," "Someone Like You," and "Set Fire to the Rain," and won six Grammy Awards in one night. She continued with *25* (2015), which sold over 3 million copies in its first week in the United States, and *30* (2021), both reaching number one in multiple countries. She won the Academy Award and Golden Globe for "Skyfall" (2012) and launched the Las Vegas residency *Weekends with Adele* beginning in 2022.

Alec Baldwin is an actor who moved from early 1980s television, including *Knots Landing*, into film with *Beetlejuice* (1988) and *The Hunt for Red October* (1990). He appeared in films including *Glengarry Glen Ross*, *The Departed*, and *Mission: Impossible – Fallout*, and voiced a lead role in *The Boss Baby* (2017), which grossed over $500 million worldwide. From 2006 to 2013 he starred in NBC's *30 Rock* as Jack Donaghy, winning two Primetime Emmy Awards, three Golden Globe Awards, and multiple Screen Actors Guild Awards. He hosted *Saturday Night Live* a record 17 times and won another Emmy Award for portraying Donald Trump. He continued working across television, film, and voice roles into the 2020s.

Alex Hormozi is an entrepreneur who left management consulting after graduating from Vanderbilt University to open a gym in 2013, scaling to multiple locations before selling his ownership interests and advising other fitness businesses. He founded Gym Launch and Prestige Labs, providing licensing, supplements, and services to gym owners internationally, and later co-founded ALAN, a customer acquisition software platform. He and his partners exited majority stakes in Gym Launch and Prestige Labs in 2021. In 2020 he co-founded Acquisition.com, investing in and advising privately held companies, focusing on service, software, and e-commerce businesses. He has published business books including *$100M Offers* and *$100M Leads* and distributes operational frameworks through digital media reaching a large global audience of entrepreneurs.

Alice Cooper is a singer and songwriter who fronted the Alice Cooper band, breaking through with *Love It to Death* (1971), *Killer* (1971), *School's Out* (1972), and the number-one album *Billion Dollar Babies* (1973). After the band split in 1975, he launched a solo career with *Welcome to My Nightmare* and went on to release more than 25 studio albums and sell over 50 million records worldwide. He returned to mainstream charts with *Trash* (1989), which included the hit single "Poison." He continued touring internationally and appeared in films and television. The original Alice Cooper band was inducted into the Rock and Roll Hall of Fame in 2011, recognizing its influence on rock performance and recording.

Allen Iverson is a basketball player who was the first overall pick in the 1996 NBA Draft and spent most of his 14-year NBA career with the Philadelphia 76ers. He won Rookie of the Year in 1997 and league MVP in 2001 while leading the 76ers to the NBA Finals that season. He won four NBA scoring titles and averaged 26.7 points, 6.2 assists, and 2.2 steals over 914 regular-season games. He played for the 76ers, Denver Nuggets, and Detroit Pistons, returning briefly to Philadelphia in 2009–10. An 11-time All-Star and three-time All-NBA First Team guard, he was inducted into the Naismith Memorial Basketball Hall of Fame in 2016.

Allie Bailey is an ultrarunner and coach who has completed more than 200 marathons and ultramarathons and recorded multiple endurance "firsts," including a 100-mile crossing of Mongolia's frozen Lake Khövsgöl and running the full length of the Panama Canal. She completed an off-road Land's End to John o'Groats route of 1,053 miles in 35 days. She founded the coaching company Ultra Awesome and won Coach of the Year at the 2024 National Running Awards. She published the memoir *There Is No Wall* and expanded into speaking, podcasts, and endurance coaching programs built around multi-day expedition running.

Amber "Mac" MacArthur is a technology host and entrepreneur who started in San Francisco and Boston during the dot-com boom, working at Razorfish and as marketing director for an e-procurement software company before returning to Canada to work as a web strategist at Microsoft. She moved into tech media, co-hosting G4TechTV Canada's *Call for Help* and later appearing on Citytv/CP24, BNN's *App Central*, and Bloomberg's *Brink*. She hosts *The Feed* and *The AmberMac Show* on SiriusXM and runs AmberMac Media Inc., producing podcasts including *The AI Effect*, *Marketing Disrupted*, and *This Is Mining*. She published *Power Friending* and co-authored *Outsmarting Your Kids Online* while keynoting conferences internationally.

Amber Valletta is a model and actress who began modeling as a teenager, landing her first *American Vogue* cover in February 1993 and appearing on the magazine's cover 17 times. She became the face of major fashion houses including Chanel, Louis Vuitton, Prada, Gucci, and Versace, and walked runway shows in Paris, Milan, London, and New York across multiple decades. In the 2000s she expanded into television and film, hosting MTV's *House of Style* and acting in projects including *Hitch*, *Transporter 2*, and the series *Revenge*. She was named to the Oklahoma Hall of Fame Class of 2024 while continuing fashion work and public advocacy tied to sustainability and industry reform.

Amy Robach is a television journalist who moved from local news in Charleston and Washington, D.C., to NBC News in 2003 as a national correspondent, later co-anchoring *Weekend Today* and serving as an MSNBC anchor. She joined ABC News in 2012 as a *Good Morning America* correspondent and became the program's news anchor in 2014. From 2018 to 2023 she co-anchored *20/20* and, beginning in 2020, hosted *Pandemic: What You Need to Know*, which evolved into *GMA3: What You Need to Know*, co-anchoring it from 2020 to 2022. After revealing a 2013 breast cancer diagnosis following an on-air mammogram, she published the New York Times bestseller *Better* and received the University of Georgia Grady College's Distinguished Achievement in Broadcasting and Cable Award.

Andrew Carnegie is an industrialist and philanthropist who emigrated from Scotland to the United States in 1848 and rose from telegraph messenger and railroad clerk to investments in iron, rail production, and oil. In the 1870s–1890s he consolidated operations into Carnegie Steel, scaling Bessemer production and vertical integration to become a leading U.S. steel supplier for rails and construction during the country's industrial expansion. He sold Carnegie Steel to J. P. Morgan in 1901 for about $480 million, a deal that helped form U.S. Steel. He then focused on philanthropy, funding more than 2,500 public libraries and endowing institutions including Carnegie Hall, the Carnegie Institution for Science, the Carnegie Endowment for International Peace, and the Carnegie Corporation of New York.

Andrew Huberman is a neuroscientist and tenured associate professor of neurobiology and ophthalmology at Stanford University School of Medicine, where he directs the Huberman Lab. He earned a B.A. at UC Santa Barbara and completed an M.A. at UC Berkeley and a Ph.D. in neuroscience at UC Davis. He conducted postdoctoral work at Stanford as a Helen Hay Whitney Postdoctoral Fellow and held a faculty position at UC San Diego before joining Stanford's faculty in 2016. His lab has published in journals including *Nature*, *Cell*, *Science*, and *Neuron* on visual circuits, regeneration, and stress-related neural pathways. His work has been recognized with the ARVO Cogan Award and the Pew Biomedical Scholar and McKnight Neuroscience Scholar awards. He hosts the *Huberman Lab* podcast, launched in 2020, focused on science-based tools for sleep, stress, and performance.

Andy Murray is a tennis player who turned professional in 2005 and won 46 ATP singles titles, including the US Open in 2012 and Wimbledon in 2013 and 2016. He reached world No. 1 in the ATP rankings in November 2016 and finished that year as the season-ending No. 1. He reached 11 Grand Slam singles finals and won 14 ATP Masters 1000 titles. He led Great Britain to the 2015 Davis Cup title. At the Olympics he became the first tennis player to win two singles gold medals, winning at London 2012 and Rio 2016. He recorded more than

700 career match wins and earned over $60 million in prize money, continuing to compete after hip resurfacing surgery in 2019.

Anerlisa Muigai is an entrepreneur and business executive, and the daughter of Keroche Breweries founders Tabitha and the late Joseph Karanja. She founded Nero Limited in 2013, launching premium bottled water brands including Executive Still Water and Life Still Water, supplying corporate clients, events, and hospitality markets in Kenya. She expanded Nero into national retail and distribution channels and was recognized as runner-up in Bizna's 2018 Young Entrepreneurs Award and received nominations in regional entrepreneurship award programs. She later paused Nero's operations and shifted into consulting and brand development while maintaining a public presence as a business leader and digital media figure.

Ann Dowsett Johnston is a journalist, author, and psychotherapist who spent decades as a magazine journalist and editor, winning multiple National Magazine Awards and serving as vice principal of McGill University. She was awarded the Atkinson Fellowship in Public Policy, producing an investigative series examining alcohol policy, gender, and public health. She published *Drink: The Intimate Relationship Between Women and Alcohol* in 2013, which was named among the year's notable books by *The Washington Post*. She later retrained as a psychotherapist and social worker, establishing a clinical practice focused on women's mental health and life transitions. She teaches writing and speaks internationally on public health, addiction, and gender-related policy issues.

Anne Hathaway is an actress who broke out in Disney's *The Princess Diaries* (2001) and its 2004 sequel, then moved into adult roles with *Brokeback Mountain* (2005) and *The Devil Wears Prada* (2006). She starred in films including *Rachel Getting Married*, *Get Smart*, *Alice in Wonderland*, *The Dark Knight Rises*, *Les Misérables*, *Interstellar*, *The Intern*, and *Ocean's 8*, with her films grossing more than $6.8 billion worldwide. She won the Academy Award, BAFTA Award, Golden Globe Award, and Screen Actors Guild Award for *Les Misérables*, and received a Primetime Emmy Award for voice work on *The Simpsons*. She continued starring in film and streaming projects into the 2020s.

Anne Lamott is an author who published her first novel, *Hard Laughter*, in 1980, followed by novels including *Rosie*, *Joe Jones*, *Crooked Little Heart*, *Blue Shoe*, and *Imperfect Birds*. She reached national prominence with the memoir *Operating Instructions: A Journal of My Son's First Year* (1993) and the writing guide *Bird by Bird: Some Instructions on Writing and Life* (1994), which became widely used by writers. She published multiple New York Times bestselling nonfiction books and essay collections on faith, recovery, and daily life. She taught writing at the University of California, Davis, and conducted workshops nationally. She received a Guggenheim Fellowship and was inducted into the California Hall of Fame in 2010.

Annie Grace is an author and entrepreneur who worked in corporate marketing, rising to senior leadership roles at a multinational company overseeing international campaigns. She left corporate leadership and self-published *This Naked Mind* in 2015, which became a bestselling book and was later republished by Penguin Random House. She founded This Naked Mind, LLC and created The Alcohol Experiment, developing online programs, podcasts, and educational resources focused on behavioral change. She expanded the company into a global digital platform offering courses, coaching, and community-based programs, reaching a large international audience through books, media, and online initiatives.

Anthony Hopkins is an actor who began on the British stage and television, winning a BAFTA TV Award for *War and Peace* and a Primetime Emmy Award for *The Bunker*. His international breakthrough came as Hannibal Lecter in *The Silence of the Lambs* (1991), which earned him the Academy Award for Best Actor. He starred in films including *The Remains of the Day*, *Nixon*, *Legends of the Fall*, and *Meet Joe Black*. He later appeared in major franchises including *Thor* and *Transformers: The Last Knight*, and portrayed Robert Ford in the HBO series *Westworld*. He won a second Academy Award for Best Actor for *The Father* (2020) at age 83, becoming the oldest Best Actor winner in Academy Awards history.

Ari Lennox is a singer and songwriter who became the first female artist signed to J. Cole's Dreamville Records in 2015. She contributed to Dreamville compilation projects including *Revenge of the Dreamers II* and the Grammy-nominated *Revenge of the Dreamers III*. Her debut studio album *Shea Butter Baby* (2019) included the platinum-certified title track featuring J. Cole and supported her first headlining Shea Butter Baby Tour. She released her second studio album *age/sex/location* in 2022 and followed with North American touring and festival appearances. Her recordings have achieved platinum certification and accumulated hundreds of millions of streams across digital platforms as she continued releasing music and performing into the 2020s.

Arthur Brooks is an economist, author, and academic who spent over a decade as a professional French horn player before earning a Ph.D. in public policy and entering academia. He published dozens of peer-reviewed articles and books including *Social Entrepreneurship*. In 2009 he became president of the American Enterprise Institute, serving until 2019 and expanding its programs and fundraising. Since 2019 he has taught at Harvard Kennedy School and Harvard Business School, where he leads research and teaching on leadership and well-being. He has authored multiple books including the New York Times bestseller *From Strength to Strength* and co-authored *Build the Life You Want* with Oprah Winfrey. He also writes a regular column for The Atlantic and speaks internationally on leadership, happiness, and public policy.

Augusten Burroughs is an author who left school after sixth grade, moved to New York City at 17, and spent over 17 years in advertising, working as a copywriter on national brands before writing full time. His first novel, *Sellevision* (2000), was followed by the memoir *Running with Scissors* (2002), a long-running New York Times bestseller adapted into a feature film. He then published *Dry* (2003), the essay collections *Magical Thinking* (2004) and *Possible Side Effects* (2006), and memoirs including *A Wolf at the Table*, *This Is How*, *Lust & Wonder*, and *Toil & Trouble*. His books have been translated into over 40 languages.

Bella Hadid is a model who signed with IMG Models in 2014 and quickly booked major runway work, including Chanel and Givenchy, before landing her first *Vogue* cover with *Vogue Turkey* (May 2016). In 2017 she set a record by appearing on five international *Vogue* September covers. She became a Dior Makeup ambassador in 2016 and fronted campaigns for brands including Bulgari, DKNY, TAG Heuer, and Max Mara. In 2021 she joined Kin Euphorics as co-founder and business partner, expanding into product and brand development while continuing high-fashion editorial, runway, and global campaign work into the 2020s.

Ben Affleck is an actor, filmmaker, producer who broke through in 1997 when he co-wrote and starred in *Good Will Hunting*, winning the Academy Award and Golden Globe for best original screenplay (with Matt Damon). He became a leading studio actor in *Armageddon* (1998), *Pearl Harbor* (2001), and *The Sum of All Fears* (2002), then moved into directing with *Gone Baby Gone* (2007) and *The Town* (2010). He directed, produced, and starred in *Argo* (2012), which won the Academy Award for best picture and earned him the DGA, Golden Globe, and BAFTA directing awards. He played Batman in *Batman v Superman* (2016) and *Justice League* (2017), with a cameo in *The Flash* (2023). In 2022 he co-founded Artists Equity and directed *Air* (2023), later producing and starring in *The Accountant 2* (2025).

Ben Harper is a singer-songwriter, guitarist who became famous in 1994 with his debut album *Welcome to the Cruel World*, establishing himself through touring and follow-up albums including *Fight for Your Mind* (1995) and *Diamonds on the Inside* (2003). He has released more than a dozen studio albums as a solo artist and collaborator, blending folk, blues, rock, soul, and reggae. He has won three Grammy Awards: best traditional soul gospel album with The Blind Boys of Alabama for *There Will Be a Light* (2004), best pop instrumental performance for "11th Commandment" (2004), and best blues album with Charlie Musselwhite for *Get Up!* (2014). He has also collaborated with artists including Mavis Staples, Natalie Maines, and Rickie Lee Jones.

Billy Joel is a singer-songwriter, pianist who gained national recognition in 1973 with his album *Piano Man*, establishing a signature song and national recognition. Between 1977 and 1983 he released *The Stranger*, *52nd Street*, *Glass Houses*, and *An Innocent Man*, producing multiple hit singles and multi-platinum albums. He has achieved 33 top 40 hits on the Billboard Hot 100, and his *Greatest Hits Volume I & Volume II* is certified over 23× platinum in the United States. His catalog has sold more than 150 million records worldwide. He has won six Grammy Awards and received the Grammy Legend Award in 1990. He was inducted into the Songwriters Hall of Fame in 1992 and the Rock and Roll Hall of Fame in 1999, and has maintained a long-running residency at Madison Square Garden since 2014.

Björn Borg is a tennis player who became widely known in the mid-1970s, winning his first French Open in 1974 and becoming world No. 1. He won 11 major singles titles, including six French Open titles and five consecutive Wimbledon championships from 1976 to 1980. He reached 16 Grand Slam singles finals and completed the French Open–Wimbledon double three straight years from 1978 to 1980. He won 66 career singles titles and compiled a 609–127 match record. He never won the U.S. Open, finishing runner-up four times. In 1979 he became the first player to earn more than $1 million in prize money in a single season. He retired in 1983 at age 26 and later served as Team Europe captain in the Laver Cup beginning in 2017.

Blac Chyna (Angela White) is a television personality, entrepreneur who broke through in the early 2010s as a video model and gained wider recognition through appearances on *Keeping Up with the Kardashians* and the reality series *Rob & Chyna* (2016). In 2014 she founded Lashed Cosmetics and opened beauty salons offering cosmetic services and retail products. She later became a top creator on OnlyFans, joining the platform in 2020 and deactivating her account in 2023. She has also pursued acting, brand partnerships, and business ventures while appearing in television and media projects. In 2023 she publicly began using her birth name, Angela White, and continued developing beauty, lifestyle, and media initiatives.

Blake Lively is an actress, entrepreneur who achieved early recognition as Serena van der Woodsen on the television series *Gossip Girl* (2007–2012). She appeared in films including *The Sisterhood of the*

Traveling Pants (2005), *The Town* (2010), *The Age of Adaline* (2015), *The Shallows* (2016), and *A Simple Favor* (2018). She founded Betty Buzz in 2021, a beverage company producing sparkling mixers, and expanded into canned cocktails with Betty Booze in 2023. She has also worked as a producer on film and television projects. In 2024 she starred in *It Ends With Us*, based on the Colleen Hoover novel, which became a major theatrical release.

Brad Pitt is an actor, producer who became known with roles in *Thelma & Louise* (1991) and *A River Runs Through It* (1992), rising to leading roles in *Se7en* (1995), *12 Monkeys* (1995), and *Fight Club* (1999). He starred in major films including *Ocean's Eleven* (2001), *Troy* (2004), *Mr. & Mrs. Smith* (2005), and *World War Z* (2013), as well as *The Curious Case of Benjamin Button* (2008), *Moneyball* (2011), and *Once Upon a Time in Hollywood* (2019). He won the Academy Award for best supporting actor for *Once Upon a Time in Hollywood*. Through Plan B Entertainment, he produced Academy Award winners for best picture including *12 Years a Slave* (2013) and *Moonlight* (2016). He has remained active in film acting and producing into the 2020s.

Bradley Cooper is an actor, filmmaker who broke through with the comedy *The Hangover* (2009), which led to two sequels and established him as a leading film actor. He previously appeared in supporting roles in *Wedding Crashers* (2005) and *Yes Man* (2008). He earned Academy Award nominations for acting in *Silver Linings Playbook* (2012), *American Hustle* (2013), and *American Sniper* (2014). He co-wrote, directed, and starred in *A Star Is Born* (2018), which received multiple Academy Award nominations and featured the Oscar-winning song "Shallow." He later co-wrote, directed, produced, and starred in *Maestro* (2023), earning additional Academy Award nominations for acting and producing. He has also produced and starred in films and remained active in directing and producing.

Brené Brown is a researcher, author who became widely known in 2010 when her TEDxHouston talk "The Power of Vulnerability" gained global attention. She served as a research professor at the University of Houston Graduate College of Social Work, studying shame, vulnerability, courage, and leadership. She has authored multiple New

York Times bestselling books, including *The Gifts of Imperfection* (2010), *Daring Greatly* (2012), *Rising Strong* (2015), *Braving the Wilderness* (2017), *Dare to Lead* (2018), and *Atlas of the Heart* (2021). She created The Daring Way, a training program based on her research. She launched the podcast *Unlocking Us* in 2020 and hosted the HBO Max series *Brené Brown: Atlas of the Heart* (2022), expanding her work into media, leadership training, and education.

Brett Favre is a football player who became the starting quarterback of the Green Bay Packers in 1992, beginning a record-setting 20-season NFL career. He played for the Atlanta Falcons, Packers, New York Jets, and Minnesota Vikings, becoming the first quarterback to surpass 70,000 passing yards, 10,000 attempts, 6,000 completions, and 500 touchdown passes. He won three consecutive AP NFL MVP awards from 1995 to 1997 and led the Packers to victory in Super Bowl XXXI and an appearance in Super Bowl XXXII. He made 297 consecutive regular-season starts and retired with 71,838 passing yards, 508 touchdowns, and 11 Pro Bowl selections. He was inducted into the Pro Football Hall of Fame in 2016.

Bruce Lee is a martial artist, actor who gained international recognition starring in Hong Kong films beginning with *The Big Boss* (1971), establishing himself as a leading martial arts film star. Born in San Francisco and raised in Hong Kong, he acted in films as a child and later moved to the United States, where he taught martial arts and developed Jeet Kune Do. He appeared on American television as Kato in *The Green Hornet* (1966–1967). He starred in *Fist of Fury* (1972), *The Way of the Dragon* (1972), and *Enter the Dragon* (1973), which became a global commercial success. His work helped expand martial arts cinema internationally. He died in 1973 at age 32, and *Enter the Dragon* was later selected for preservation in the U.S. National Film Registry.

Calvin Harris is a DJ, producer, songwriter who entered the public spotlight with his debut album *I Created Disco* (2007), which produced UK top 10 singles including "Acceptable in the 80s." His album *18 Months* (2012) generated eight UK top 10 singles, setting a record for a studio album by a solo artist. He achieved global success with songs including "We Found Love," "Feel So Close," "Summer," and "This Is What You Came For." He became the first artist to reach one billion streams on Spotify as a lead artist. He held major Las Vegas DJ residencies and was named Forbes' highest-paid DJ for six consecutive years from 2013 to 2018. He has won Grammy and BRIT Awards and continued releasing hit singles and collaborations into the 2020s.

Cara Delevingne is a model, actress who rose to prominence after signing with Storm Management in 2009 and gaining international attention through Burberry campaigns and runway work beginning in 2011. She won model of the year at the British Fashion Awards in 2012 and 2014 and appeared in campaigns and shows for brands including Chanel, Fendi, Dolce & Gabbana, and Victoria's Secret. She transitioned into acting with a role in *Anna Karenina* (2012) and later starred in *Paper Towns* (2015), *Suicide Squad* (2016), and *Valerian and the City of a Thousand Planets* (2017). She also appeared in the television series *Carnival Row* (2019–2023) and *Only Murders in the Building* (2022), continuing work in film, television, and fashion.

Caroline Knapp is a journalist, author who established her career in Boston journalism before gaining national recognition as a memoirist. She wrote for the *Providence Eagle* and *Boston Business Magazine*, then served as a columnist and editor at the *Boston Phoenix* from 1988 to 1995, where her "Out There" column inspired her first book, *Alice K.'s Guide to Life* (1994). She achieved wide attention with *Drinking: A Love Story* (1996), which spent weeks on *The New York Times* bestseller list. She later authored *Pack of Two* (1998), examining human–dog relationships. Before her death in 2002, she completed *Appetites: Why Women Want*, published posthumously in 2003, along with the essay collection *The Merry Recluse*, cementing her legacy in memoir and cultural criticism.

Carrie Bates (Carrie Steinseifer-Bates) is a swimmer who achieved international success representing the United States in the 1980s. She won Olympic gold medals in relay events at the 1984 Los Angeles Olympics and earned additional international gold medals at the 1987 Pan American Games and 1989 Pan Pacific Championships. She trained with West Valley Aquatics and competed collegiately at the University of Texas, contributing to national championship teams. After retiring from competitive swimming, she later competed in endurance events including Ironman triathlons. She has also worked in advocacy and leadership roles with organizations including Hazelden Betty Ford Foundation and Caron Treatment Centers.

Casey Neistat is a filmmaker, youtuber who gained early attention in 2003 with the viral short film "iPod's Dirty Secret," criticizing Apple's iPod battery replacement policies. In 2008 HBO acquired and aired *The Neistat Brothers*, an autobiographical television series he created with his brother. He launched his YouTube channel in 2010 and built a large audience through daily vlogs and filmmaking projects. In 2015 he co-founded the social media app Beme, which was acquired by CNN in 2016. He later returned to independent filmmaking, brand collaborations, and online video, continuing to produce content across YouTube and other platforms into the 2020s.

Cat Marnell is a writer, journalist who gained national recognition as beauty and health editor at xoJane, where her first-person columns about fashion, nightlife, and personal experiences drew a wide readership. She previously worked in beauty departments at publications including *NYLON*, *Teen Vogue*, *Glamour*, and *Lucky*. In 2012 she left xoJane and later wrote the "Amphetamine Logic" column for Vice. Her memoir, *How to Murder Your Life* (2017), became a New York Times bestseller and recounts her career in New York media and personal life. She has continued writing essays, journalism, and subscription-based newsletter content, maintaining a presence in independent media and publishing.

Catherine Gray is a journalist, author who built her career writing and editing for British women's magazines including *Cosmopolitan*, *Glamour*, *Eve*, and *Fabulous*, before moving into freelance journalism. She gained wider recognition with her book *The Unexpected Joy of Being Sober* (2017), which became a Sunday Times bestseller. She later published related titles including *The Unexpected Joy of Being Sober Journal*, *The Unexpected Joy of Being Single* (2019), and *The Unexpected Joy of the Ordinary* (2023). Her work led to podcast appearances, media contributions, and co-creating the "Sober Spring" campaign with Alcohol Change UK. She has continued writing books and speaking about habits, behavior, and lifestyle topics into the 2020s.

CC Sabathia is a baseball pitcher who debuted with the Cleveland Indians in 2001 at age 20 and became one of the American League's top starters. He won the AL Cy Young Award in 2007 after leading the league in innings pitched. Traded to the Milwaukee Brewers in 2008, he led them to their first postseason appearance since 1982, then signed with the New York Yankees and helped win the 2009 World Series. He led the AL in wins in 2009 and 2010 and reached 3,000 strikeouts and 251 career wins. He retired in 2019 after 19 seasons and was elected to the National Baseball Hall of Fame in 2025.

Celeste Yvonne is an author, speaker who gained national attention writing essays on motherhood, parenting, and modern family life, featured by outlets including *The Washington Post*, *Today*, and Refinery29. She worked for more than two decades in corporate communications and marketing while building an online writing career. She co-founded the Sober Mom Squad, an online community, and later published *It's Not About the Wine: The Loaded Truth Behind Mommy Wine Culture* (2023). She has expanded her work through media appearances, speaking engagements, and coaching, and publishes ongoing writing through her Substack newsletter, *The Ultimate Mom Challenge*, focusing on parenting, mental load, and lifestyle topics.

Charlie Kirk is a political activist, media host who founded Turning Point USA in 2012 at age 18, building a national conservative student organization focused on free markets and limited government. He expanded Turning Point USA into a nationwide campus network and launched *The Charlie Kirk Show*, distributed across radio, podcast, and digital platforms. He authored books including *Time for a Turning Point* (2016) and *The MAGA Doctrine* (2020), addressing political activism and conservative ideas. On September 10, 2025, he was assassinated by a sniper while speaking at Utah Valley University in Orem, Utah, ending his career at age 31

Charlie Sheen is an actor who gained national recognition in the 1980s with roles in *Red Dawn* (1984), *Platoon* (1986), and *Wall Street* (1987). He later starred in comedies including *Major League* (1989) and *Hot Shots!* (1991) and its sequel *Hot Shots! Part Deux* (1993). He appeared in films including *Being John Malkovich* (1999). On television, he replaced Michael J. Fox on *Spin City* (2000–2002), winning a Golden Globe Award in 2002. He starred in *Two and a Half Men* (2003–2011), earning multiple Emmy and Golden Globe nominations. He received a star on the Hollywood Walk of Fame in 1994 and has continued acting in television and film projects.

Chelsea Handler is a comedian, television host, author who rose to prominence hosting the late-night talk show *Chelsea Lately* on E! from 2007 to 2014. She previously appeared on television in *Girls Behaving Badly* (2002–2005) and hosted *The Chelsea Handler Show* (2006). She has published multiple New York Times bestselling books, including *My Horizontal Life* (2005), *Chelsea Chelsea Bang Bang* (2010), *Lies That Chelsea Handler Told Me* (2011), and *Uganda Be Kidding Me* (2014). NBC adapted her book into the sitcom *Are You There, Chelsea?* (2012). She later hosted the Netflix talk series *Chelsea* (2016–2017) and has continued releasing stand-up specials, touring, and publishing books into the 2020s.

Chris Herren is a basketball player, author who achieved early recognition as a high school standout at Durfee High School in Fall River, Massachusetts, before playing college basketball at Boston College and Fresno State, where he earned first-team All-WAC honors. He was selected in the 1999 NBA draft and played for the Denver Nuggets and Boston Celtics from 1999 to 2001. He continued his professional career in international leagues including Italy, Turkey, China, and Germany, scoring 63 points in a game for the Beijing Ducks. He founded the Herren Project in 2011, a nonprofit providing education and support services. He authored the memoir *Basketball Junkie* and was the subject of the ESPN documentary *Unguarded*.

Chris Williamson is a media host, entrepreneur who first reached public visibility as a contestant on the debut season of *Love Island* (UK) in 2015, then transitioned from nightlife promotion into digital media.

In 2018 he launched the long-form interview podcast *Modern Wisdom*, releasing frequent episodes and building a catalogue exceeding 900 interviews. The show features conversations with academics, authors, athletes, and entrepreneurs and is distributed across podcast platforms and YouTube, where it has accumulated a global audience in the millions by the mid-2020s. Alongside his media work, he co-founded the functional beverage brand Neutonic and has spoken publicly about productivity, attention, and modern culture, positioning *Modern Wisdom* as a forum for extended, research-driven discussion.

Chrissy Teigen is a model, television personality, entrepreneur who rose to prominence after appearing in the *Sports Illustrated Swimsuit Issue*, where she was named Rookie of the Year in 2010 and later appeared on multiple covers, including the 50th anniversary issue in 2014. She co-hosted the television series *Lip Sync Battle* from 2015 to 2019 and appeared as a judge on competition shows including *Bring the Funny* (2019). She launched the food brand Cravings, beginning with her bestselling cookbook *Cravings: Recipes for All the Food You Want to Eat* (2016), followed by additional cookbooks and product lines. She expanded Cravings into cookware and packaged foods sold through national retailers including Target, building a lifestyle and consumer products business.

Christina Ricci is an actress who came to prominence as Wednesday Addams in *The Addams Family* (1991) and *Addams Family Values* (1993), after making her film debut in *Mermaids* (1990). She starred in films including *Casper* (1995), *Now and Then* (1995), *The Ice Storm* (1997), *The Opposite of Sex* (1998), *Sleepy Hollow* (1999), and *Monster* (2003), earning a Golden Globe nomination for *The Opposite of Sex*. She made her Broadway debut in *Time Stands Still* (2010). On television, she received Emmy nominations for *Grey's Anatomy* (2006) and *Yellowjackets* (2022), and joined the cast of Netflix's *Wednesday* (2022). She has also served as a national spokesperson for RAINN.

Clare Pooley is an author, former advertising executive who built a career in advertising, rising to managing partner at J. Walter Thompson and working on global accounts including Nestlé, Shell, Unilever, and Rolex. She later began the blog *Mummy Was a Secret*

Drinker, which led to her memoir *The Sober Diaries* (2017), published internationally. Her debut novel, *The Authenticity Project* (2020), became a New York Times bestseller, was translated into multiple languages, and won the Romantic Novelists' Association Debut Romantic Novel Award. She has since published novels including *The People on Platform 5* (2022) and *How to Age Disgracefully* (2024), establishing her career in contemporary fiction.

Colin Farrell is an actor who established his film career with roles in *Tigerland* (2000), *Minority Report* (2002), *Phone Booth* (2002), *S.W.A.T.* (2003), and *Miami Vice* (2006). He earned critical recognition for performances in *In Bruges* (2008), winning the Golden Globe Award for best actor, and later starred in *The Lobster* (2015) and *The Banshees of Inisherin* (2022), receiving an Academy Award nomination and winning another Golden Globe. He also appeared in franchise films including *Fantastic Beasts and Where to Find Them* (2016), *Dumbo* (2019), and portrayed the Penguin in *The Batman* (2022) and the HBO series *The Penguin* (2024). His work has earned multiple Golden Globe, SAG, and Critics Choice awards across film and television.

Colin Plume is an entrepreneur, author who founded Noble Gold Investments in 2016, a company specializing in precious metals and self-directed IRA accounts. He previously worked in property insurance and commercial real estate, advising investors on asset protection and risk management. Through Noble Gold, he expanded into precious metals investment services and later launched related ventures including the digital asset platform My Digital Money and the human resources firm GuardianHR. He authored the investing book *Silver Is the New Oil* (2024), which became an Amazon bestseller and led to media appearances discussing precious metals, inflation, and alternative investments. His work focuses on investment education and alternative asset strategies.

Craig Ferguson is a comedian, television host, author who became widely known in stand-up comedy and British television before gaining U.S. visibility on ABC's *Maybe This Time* (1995). He reached a wider audience playing Nigel Wick on *The Drew Carey Show* from 1996 to

2004. He hosted *The Late Late Show with Craig Ferguson* on CBS from 2005 to 2014, producing more than 2,000 episodes. He wrote and directed *I'll Be There* (2003) and co-wrote the film *Saving Grace* (2000). He authored books including *Between the Bridge and the River* (2006) and *American on Purpose* (2009). He later hosted *Celebrity Name Game*, winning Daytime Emmy Awards for outstanding game show host in 2015 and 2016.

Cristiano Ronaldo is a soccer player who rose to international prominence after joining Manchester United in 2003, where he won three Premier League titles and the 2008 UEFA Champions League. He won his first Ballon d'Or in 2008 and transferred to Real Madrid in 2009, scoring 450 goals in 438 appearances and winning four Champions League titles. He joined Juventus in 2018, winning two Serie A titles, returned to Manchester United in 2021, and signed with Al Nassr in 2023. With Portugal, he won UEFA Euro 2016 and the 2019 Nations League. He became the first men's player to reach 200 international caps and has scored over 100 international goals, maintaining a professional career across more than two decades.

Daniel Radcliffe is an actor who became internationally known portraying Harry Potter in eight films released between 2001 and 2011. He began acting as a child and appeared in stage productions including *Equus* in London and on Broadway in 2007. He later starred on Broadway in *How to Succeed in Business Without Really Trying* (2011), *The Cripple of Inishmaan* (2014), and *Merrily We Roll Along* (2023), winning the Tony Award for best featured actor in a musical. His film work includes *Swiss Army Man* (2016), *Now You See Me 2* (2016), and *Escape from Pretoria* (2020). He has also appeared in television series including *Miracle Workers*, maintaining an active career across film, television, and theater..

Darren Waller is a football player who entered the NFL as a sixth-round draft pick by the Baltimore Ravens in 2015 after playing college football at Georgia Tech. He transitioned from wide receiver to tight end and later joined the Oakland Raiders, where he became a leading receiver. In 2019 he recorded 90 receptions for 1,145 yards and was selected to the Pro Bowl. He followed with 107 receptions, 1,196 yards, and nine touchdowns in 2020, earning a second Pro Bowl selection. He later played for the New York Giants after being traded in 2023. Over his NFL career, he recorded hundreds of receptions and thousands of receiving yards, establishing himself as a top tight end.

Darryl Strawberry is a baseball player who debuted with the New York Mets in 1983, winning National League Rookie of the Year and beginning an eight-year All-Star streak. He helped the Mets win the 1986 World Series, joined the 30–30 club in 1987, and led the National League in home runs in 1988. He played 17 Major League seasons with the Mets, Dodgers, Giants, and Yankees, hitting 335 career home runs and recording over 1,000 RBIs. He won four World Series titles, including one with the Mets and three with the Yankees. After retiring, he became a minister and co-founded Strawberry Ministries, focusing on faith-based outreach and public speaking.

Dave Mustaine is a guitarist, singer, songwriter who co-founded Metallica in 1981 and served as its original lead guitarist before departing in 1983. He then formed Megadeth, where he became the frontman and primary songwriter, helping establish the band as part of thrash metal's "Big Four" alongside Metallica, Slayer, and Anthrax. Megadeth has released sixteen studio albums and sold over 50 million records worldwide. The band's album *Countdown to Extinction* (1992) debuted at No. 2 on the Billboard 200. Mustaine won a Grammy Award for best metal performance in 2017 for Megadeth's song "Dystopia." He has continued recording, touring internationally, and overseeing Megadeth's releases across more than four decades.

David Furnish is a filmmaker, producer, executive who co-founded Rocket Pictures with Elton John in 1996 and has produced and directed film and television projects. He directed the documentary *Elton John: Tantrums & Tiaras* (1997) and produced films including *Women Talking Dirty* (1999), *It's a Boy Girl Thing* (2006), *Gnomeo & Juliet* (2011), *Sherlock Gnomes* (2018), and the biographical film *Rocketman* (2019). He has served in executive roles overseeing media, entertainment, and business operations connected to Elton John's career. He is chairman of the Elton John AIDS Foundation, supporting international HIV/AIDS programs and charitable initiatives.

David Goggins is an endurance athlete, author who served in the U.S. Navy and completed SEAL training, U.S. Army Ranger School, and Air Force Tactical Air Controller training. After military service including deployments with SEAL Team 5, he became an ultramarathon runner and endurance competitor, completing dozens of ultra-distance races such as the Badwater 135 and Ultraman World Championship. In 2013 he set a Guinness World Record by performing 4,030 pull-ups in 17 hours. He later authored the memoir *Can't Hurt Me* (2018), which became a bestseller and expanded his career into public speaking and coaching focused on mental resilience and physical performance.

David Letterman is a television host, comedian, producer who established his late-night career with *Late Night with David Letterman* on NBC (1982–1993) and continued with *Late Show with David Letterman* on CBS (1993–2015). Through his production company Worldwide Pants, he produced his own programs and additional television projects. He hosted more than 6,000 episodes across both series, introducing recurring segments including Top Ten Lists and Stupid Pet Tricks. He surpassed Johnny Carson in total number of late-night broadcasts as a host. His shows received more than 100 Emmy nominations and multiple wins. After retiring from network late night, he returned as host of the interview series *My Next Guest Needs No Introduction with David Letterman* on Netflix.

Dax Shepard is an actor, filmmaker, podcast host who first gained national exposure on MTV's *Punk'd* (2003). He appeared in films including *Without a Paddle* (2004), *Zathura* (2005), *Employee of the Month* (2006), *Idiocracy* (2006), and *Baby Mama* (2008). He starred as Crosby Braverman on NBC's *Parenthood* from 2010 to 2015 and directed episodes of the series. He wrote, directed, and starred in the films *Hit and Run* (2012) and *CHiPs* (2017). In 2018 he launched the podcast *Armchair Expert*, featuring interviews with actors, authors, and public figures, which became one of the most-listened-to podcasts across major platforms and expanded into live tours and additional podcast series.

Demi Lovato is a singer, songwriter, actor who rose to prominence through Disney Channel projects including *Camp Rock* (2008) and the series *Sonny with a Chance* (2009–2011), after early work on *Barney & Friends*. She launched a recording career with *Don't Forget* (2008) and released multiple albums that reached the top five of the Billboard 200, including *Here We Go Again* (2009), *Unbroken* (2011), *Demi* (2013), *Confident* (2015), and *Tell Me You Love Me* (2017). Her album *Confident* earned a Grammy nomination for best pop vocal album. She released the documentary series *Demi Lovato: Dancing with the Devil* (2021) and continued recording and performing, maintaining a music and television career spanning more than a decade.

Demi Moore is an actor, producer who established his career with roles in 1980s films including *St. Elmo's Fire* (1985) and achieved major commercial success starring in *Ghost* (1990), one of the highest-grossing films of its year. She starred in *A Few Good Men* (1992) and *Indecent Proposal* (1993), continuing a run of leading roles in major studio productions. In 1996 she received a reported $12.5 million salary for *Striptease*, one of the highest salaries paid to an actress at the time. She later starred in *G.I. Jane* (1997) and continued working in film and television. She published the memoir *Inside Out* (2019), which became a New York Times bestseller.

Denzel Washington is an actor, director, producer who gained national visibility on the television series *St. Elsewhere* (1982–1988) before achieving film success with *Glory* (1989), winning the Academy Award for best supporting actor. He starred in films including *Malcolm X* (1992), earning an Academy Award nomination, and later won best actor for *Training Day* (2001). His other major films include *Philadelphia* (1993), *Remember the Titans* (2000), and *The Equalizer* series. On stage, he starred in the Broadway revival of *Fences* (2010), winning a Tony Award, and later directed and starred in the film adaptation *Fences* (2016). He has maintained a leading career across film, theater, and producing for more than four decades.

Dick Van Dyke is an actor, comedian, singer, dancer who rose to prominence starring in the Broadway musical *Bye Bye Birdie* (1960–1961), winning a Tony Award. He gained national fame as Rob Petrie on *The Dick Van Dyke Show* (1961–1966), earning multiple Emmy Awards. He starred in films including *Mary Poppins* (1964) and *Chitty Chitty Bang Bang* (1968), and received a Grammy Award as part of the *Mary Poppins* soundtrack. He later starred in the television series *Diagnosis Murder* (1993–2001). Over his career, he has won six Emmy Awards, a Tony Award, and a Grammy Award, and received Kennedy Center Honors and induction into the Television Hall of Fame.

Doc Gooden is a baseball player who debuted with the New York Mets in 1984, winning National League Rookie of the Year. In 1985 he won the Cy Young Award and the pitching Triple Crown with a 24–4 record, 1.53 ERA, and 268 strikeouts, becoming the youngest 20-game winner in Major League Baseball history. He helped the Mets win the 1986 World Series and later won championships with the New York Yankees in 1996 and 2000. He pitched a no-hitter for the Yankees in 1996. Over 16 seasons with five teams, he recorded 194 wins and 2,293 strikeouts. In 2024 the Mets retired his number 16, honoring his career achievements.

Doechii is a rapper, singer, songwriter who built her early career releasing music independently on SoundCloud before gaining viral attention with the song "Yucky Blucky Fruitcake" in 2020. She signed with Top Dawg Entertainment in 2022, becoming the label's first female rapper, and released singles including "Persuasive" and the project *She / Her / Black Bitch*. Her single "What It Is (Block Boy)" entered the Billboard Hot 100 in 2023. She released the mixtape *Alligator Bites Never Heal* (2024), which reached No. 2 on Billboard's Top Rap Albums chart and earned a Grammy Award. Her music has charted across Billboard rankings, establishing her presence in mainstream hip-hop and pop.

Donald Trump is a real estate developer, television personality, politician who became president of the Trump Organization in 1971, expanding its real estate portfolio with projects including Trump Tower in New York and casino and hotel developments in Atlantic City. He gained national media prominence as host of the reality television series *The Apprentice* from 2004 to 2015. He was elected the 45th president of the United States in 2016 and served from 2017 to 2021.

He was elected again in 2024 and became the 47th president, returning to office in January 2025. His career has spanned business, television, and national politics over more than five decades.

Dr. Phil McGraw is a psychologist, television host, author who co-founded Courtroom Sciences, Inc. in 1989, providing trial consulting services that led to regular appearances on *The Oprah Winfrey Show* in the late 1990s. In 2002 he launched the syndicated television program *Dr. Phil*, which ran for more than 20 seasons and became one of the most widely viewed daytime talk shows. He has written multiple books, including several New York Times bestsellers. He co-founded the telehealth company Doctor On Demand in 2012, expanding access to medical and mental health services through digital platforms. His career has spanned psychology, publishing, television, and healthcare entrepreneurship.

Drew Barrymore is an actor, producer, television host who first gained attention as a child starring in *E.T. the Extra-Terrestrial* (1982). She later starred in films including *The Wedding Singer* (1998), *Never Been Kissed* (1999), and *50 First Dates* (2004). In 1995 she co-founded Flower Films with Nancy Juvonen, producing projects including *Charlie's Angels* (2000) and *Charlie's Angels: Full Throttle* (2003). She won a Golden Globe Award and a Screen Actors Guild Award for *Grey Gardens* (2009). Since 2020 she has hosted the syndicated daytime program *The Drew Barrymore Show* and won the Daytime Emmy Award for outstanding daytime talk series host in 2025.

Ed Sheeran is a singer-songwriter, guitarist who achieved early recognition with his debut album + (2011), which reached No. 1 in the UK and introduced the single "The A Team." His follow-up albums × (2014) and ÷ (2017) topped charts worldwide, with "Shape of You" becoming one of the best-selling singles globally and among the most-streamed songs in digital history. His ÷ Tour (2017–2019) became the highest-grossing concert tour at the time. He later released = (2021), - (2023), and *Autumn Variations* (2023), all reaching major international charts. He has won multiple Grammy Awards, BRIT Awards, and Ivor Novello Awards during a recording career spanning more than a decade.

Eliud Kipchoge is a long-distance runner who became widely known after winning the 5,000 meters at the World Championships in 2003 and earning Olympic silver (2004) and bronze (2008). He moved to marathon racing in 2013, winning his debut in Hamburg and later victories at major races including the Berlin Marathon and London Marathon. He won Olympic marathon gold medals at Rio 2016 and Tokyo 2020. He set marathon world records of 2:01:39 in 2018 and 2:01:09 in 2022, the latter becoming the official world record at the time. In 2019 he ran 1:59:40 at the INEOS 1:59 Challenge, completing the marathon distance in under two hours in a non-record-eligible event.

Elizabeth Vargas is a television journalist who gained national recognition after joining NBC News in 1993 as a correspondent for *Dateline NBC* and other programs. She moved to ABC News in 1996, serving as a correspondent and later anchor for *20/20* and *Primetime*. She briefly co-anchored *World News Tonight* in 2005–2006 and won an Emmy Award for news coverage during her career. After leaving ABC News in 2018, she hosted investigative and crime programs including *A&E Investigates* and *America's Most Wanted*. In 2023 she became host of the nightly program *Elizabeth Vargas Reports* on NewsNation, continuing her work in national television journalism.

Elle MacPherson is a model, entrepreneur, actor who achieved international recognition through fashion modeling and appeared on the cover of the *Sports Illustrated Swimsuit Issue* five times between 1986 and 1996. She expanded into business by launching Elle Macpherson Intimates in 1990 in partnership with Bendon, building a global lingerie brand. She later founded Elle Macpherson Inc., managing licensing and brand ventures across fashion and lifestyle products. She co-founded the wellness company WelleCo in 2014, developing plant-based supplement products sold internationally. Her career has included modeling, acting roles in film and television, and leadership in consumer product businesses.

Ellie Goulding is a singer-songwriter who became widely known after winning the BBC Sound of 2010 poll and releasing her debut album

Lights (2010), which reached No. 1 on the UK Albums Chart. The reissue *Bright Lights* included the single "Lights," which reached No. 2 on the Billboard Hot 100. She released subsequent albums including *Halcyon* (2012), *Delirium* (2015), *Brightest Blue* (2020), and *Higher Than Heaven* (2023), producing singles such as "Burn" and "Love Me Like You Do." She has earned multiple UK No. 1 albums and won BRIT Awards, maintaining an international recording career across more than a decade.

Elsa Hosk is a model, entrepreneur who entered international fashion after working in Sweden and moving to New York to pursue modeling full-time. She became a Victoria's Secret Angel in 2015 after appearing in the Victoria's Secret Fashion Show for several years and wore the Victoria's Secret Fantasy Bra in 2018. She has appeared in campaigns for brands including Guess, H&M, and CoverGirl, and on international magazine covers. In 2022 she founded the fashion label Helsa Studio, serving as creative director and launching collections through retail platforms including Revolve and FWRD. Her career spans fashion modeling and business ventures in apparel.

Elton John is a singer, songwriter, pianist who achieved international success with his self-titled album *Elton John* (1970) and subsequent releases including *Honky Château* (1972) and *Goodbye Yellow Brick Road* (1973). He recorded seven consecutive No. 1 albums on the U.S. Billboard chart between 1972 and 1975. His hit songs include "Your Song," "Rocket Man," and "Candle in the Wind 1997." He has sold more than 300 million records worldwide and performed thousands of concerts internationally. His Farewell Yellow Brick Road tour concluded in 2023. He has won multiple Grammy Awards, an Academy Award, a Tony Award, and an Emmy Award, achieving EGOT status.

Eminem is a rapper, songwriter, producer who achieved success with his major-label debut *The Slim Shady LP* (1999), which won a Grammy Award. He followed with *The Marshall Mathers LP* (2000) and *The Eminem Show* (2002), both of which topped charts internationally and became among the best-selling rap albums. He starred in the film *8 Mile* (2002) and performed "Lose Yourself," which won the Academy Award for best original song. He released multiple No. 1 albums on the

Billboard 200, including *Relapse* (2009) and *Recovery* (2010). His recordings have sold hundreds of millions of copies worldwide, establishing a long-running career in hip-hop and popular music.

Enes Kanter Freedom is a basketball player, activist who entered the NBA as the third overall pick in the 2011 draft by the Utah Jazz. He played 11 NBA seasons with teams including the Jazz, Thunder, Knicks, Trail Blazers, and Celtics, averaging double-digit points and contributing as a center. He reached the Western Conference finals with the Oklahoma City Thunder in 2016. In 2021 he became a U.S. citizen and legally changed his name to Enes Kanter Freedom. He has also been active in public advocacy on international human rights issues.

Eric Clapton is a guitarist, singer, songwriter who gained recognition in the 1960s performing with the Yardbirds, John Mayall's Bluesbreakers, and the band Cream. He later formed Derek and the Dominos, recording the song "Layla," and launched a solo career with albums including *461 Ocean Boulevard* (1974) and *Slowhand* (1977). His live album *Unplugged* (1992) became one of the best-selling live albums and included "Tears in Heaven." He has won 18 Grammy Awards and has been inducted into the Rock and Roll Hall of Fame three times: as a member of the Yardbirds, Cream, and as a solo artist. His career has spanned multiple decades in rock and blues music.

Ewan McGregor is an actor who gained emerged as a leading figure after starring in *Shallow Grave* (1994) and *Trainspotting* (1996). He became widely known for portraying Obi-Wan Kenobi in the *Star Wars* prequel trilogy beginning with *The Phantom Menace* (1999). He appeared in films including *Moulin Rouge!* (2001), *Big Fish* (2003), and *The Ghost Writer* (2010). He won a Golden Globe Award for his dual role in the television series *Fargo* (2017) and a Primetime Emmy Award for portraying Halston in the miniseries *Halston* (2021). He reprised Obi-Wan Kenobi in the Disney+ series *Obi-Wan Kenobi* (2022), continuing his work across film and television.

F. Scott Fitzgerald is a novelist, short-story writer who rose to prominence with his debut novel *This Side of Paradise* (1920), which became a bestseller and established his literary career. He followed with *The Beautiful and Damned* (1922) and published numerous short stories in national magazines. His novel *The Great Gatsby* (1925) later became widely studied and recognized as a major work of American fiction. He published *Tender Is the Night* (1934) and moved to Hollywood in 1937 to work as a screenwriter. At the time of his death in 1940, he had completed four novels and written more than 150 short stories. His unfinished novel *The Last Tycoon* was published posthumously in 1941

Florence Welch is a singer, songwriter who became widely known as the lead vocalist of Florence + the Machine, formed in London in 2007 with Isabella Summers. The band's debut album *Lungs* (2009) reached No. 1 on the UK Albums Chart and won the Brit Award for best British album. Subsequent albums including *Ceremonials* (2011), *How Big, How Blue, How Beautiful* (2015), *High as Hope* (2018), and *Dance Fever* (2022) achieved major chart success internationally. Her singles include "Dog Days Are Over," "Shake It Out," and "Spectrum (Say My Name)." She published the lyric collection *Useless Magic* in 2018, expanding her work beyond recorded music.

Friedrich Nietzsche is a philosopher, classical scholar who became a professor at the University of Basel in 1869 before resigning in 1879 due to health problems. He published *The Birth of Tragedy* (1872), followed by *Human, All Too Human* (1878). His later works included *The Gay Science* (1882), *Thus Spoke Zarathustra* (1883–1885), *Beyond Good and Evil* (1886), and *On the Genealogy of Morals* (1887), where he introduced ideas including the Übermensch and critiques of morality. After a mental collapse in 1889, he did not publish further works. He died in 1900, and his writings became widely studied in philosophy and intellectual history.

Gareth Bale is a soccer player who rose to international prominence at Tottenham Hotspur before transferring to Real Madrid in 2013 for a then world-record salary. He played nine seasons with Real Madrid, winning five UEFA Champions League titles and multiple domestic trophies, and scored in the 2014 Copa del Rey final and the 2018 Champions League final. He later returned to Tottenham on loan and finished his club career with Los Angeles FC, winning the MLS Cup in 2022. He earned more than 110 caps for Wales, became the nation's all-time leading scorer, and represented Wales at UEFA Euro 2016, Euro 2020, and the 2022 FIFA World Cup. He retired from professional soccer in 2023.

Gary Oldman is an actor, filmmaker who gained early recognition portraying Sid Vicious in *Sid and Nancy* (1986) and Joe Orton in *Prick Up Your Ears* (1987). He later appeared in films including *JFK* (1991), *Bram Stoker's Dracula* (1992), *Léon: The Professional* (1994), and *The Fifth Element* (1997). He reached wider audiences as Sirius Black in the *Harry Potter* series (2004–2011) and Commissioner Gordon in Christopher Nolan's *Dark Knight* trilogy (2005–2012). He starred in *Tinker Tailor Soldier Spy* (2011), *Darkest Hour* (2017), and *Mank* (2020), winning the Academy Award for Best Actor for *Darkest Hour*. Beginning in 2022, he starred as Jackson Lamb in the Apple TV+ series *Slow Horses*, earning award nominations.

Gary Vaynerchuk is an entrepreneur, investor, media executive who expanded his family's New Jersey liquor store into Wine Library, growing it into a major e-commerce retailer and launching the video series *Wine Library TV* in 2006. In 2009 he co-founded the digital advertising agency VaynerMedia, later part of the holding company VaynerX, serving global corporate clients. He became an early investor in technology companies including Facebook, Twitter, Uber, and Snapchat, and co-founded businesses including Resy and Empathy Wines, both later acquired. He has authored multiple New York Times bestselling books and built a large online audience through social media, podcasts, and speaking. In 2021 he launched VeeFriends, an NFT-based entertainment and collectibles brand that expanded into events, licensing, and media projects.

Gavin Newsom is a politician, businessman who became mayor of San Francisco in 2004 after serving on the city's Parking and Traffic Commission and Board of Supervisors. In 2004 he directed the city to issue marriage licenses to same-sex couples, prompting legal challenges and national attention. He served as mayor until 2011, when he was elected lieutenant governor of California, holding that office until 2019. He was elected governor of California in 2018 and reelected in 2022, and he survived a recall election in 2021. As governor, he has signed legislation on climate policy, gun regulation, healthcare access, and housing, and has overseen California's response to major wildfires, drought, and the COVID-19 pandemic.

George W. Bush is a politician, businessman who became governor of Texas in 1995 after prior work in the oil industry and ownership of the Texas Rangers baseball team. He was elected the 43rd president of the United States in 2000 and served two terms from 2001 to 2009. During his presidency he signed tax cuts and the No Child Left Behind Act, and after the September 11, 2001 attacks he established the Department of Homeland Security and authorized military operations in Afghanistan and Iraq. He also signed the Medicare Modernization Act creating Medicare Part D and approved the Troubled Asset Relief Program during the 2008 financial crisis. After leaving office, he remained active in public service through his presidential center and policy initiatives.

Gerard Butler is an actor, producer who entered film acting in the late 1990s after training as a lawyer, appearing in *Mrs. Brown* (1997) and *Tomorrow Never Dies* (1997). He gained recognition with the television film *Attila* (2001) and starred in *The Phantom of the Opera* (2004). He became widely known for portraying King Leonidas in *300* (2006). He later starred in action films including *Law Abiding Citizen* (2009) and the *Has Fallen* series, beginning with *Olympus Has Fallen* (2013), and voiced Stoick in the *How to Train Your Dragon* film trilogy (2010–2019). He has also appeared in romantic comedies and thrillers and continued leading films including *Plane* (2023) and *Den of Thieves 2: Pantera* (2025).

Gillian Jacobs is an actor, director who gained national recognition starring as Britta Perry on the NBC and Yahoo! series *Community* (2009–2015). She later starred as Mickey Dobbs on the Netflix series *Love* (2016–2018) and appeared in television and streaming projects including *Girls* and the animated series *Invincible*. Her film roles include *Life Partners* (2014), *Don't Think Twice* (2016), *I Used to Go Here* (2020), and the *Fear Street* trilogy (2021). She made her directing debut with the documentary short *The Queen of Code* (2015) and later directed the documentary feature *More Than Robots* (2022). She has continued working across television, film, voice acting, and directing into the 2020s.

Gisele Bündchen is a model, entrepreneur who rose to international prominence in the late 1990s after appearing in major runway shows and fashion campaigns. She appeared on numerous international Vogue covers and worked as a Victoria's Secret Angel from 1999 to 2006. She became one of the highest-paid models globally and expanded into business with ventures including Gisele Bündchen Intimates and skincare and lifestyle collaborations. She has also served as a United Nations Environment Programme Goodwill Ambassador since 2009, supporting environmental initiatives including rainforest conservation. She has remained active in fashion, business, and environmental advocacy into the 2020s.

Glennon Doyle is an author, activist who first gained attention after launching the blog Momastery in 2009 and publishing the memoir *Carry On, Warrior* (2013). Her memoir *Love Warrior* (2016) was selected for Oprah's Book Club and debuted at No. 1 on the New York Times bestseller list. Her book *Untamed* (2020) also became a No. 1 New York Times bestseller and expanded her audience. In 2012 she founded Together Rising, a nonprofit organization that raised tens of millions of dollars to support people in crisis before concluding operations in 2024. Beginning in 2021 she co-hosted the podcast *We Can Do Hard Things*, which became a widely distributed interview and discussion show.

Grant Cardone is an entrepreneur, author who established his career in sales training after working in automotive sales and consulting. He founded Cardone Training Technologies and Cardone University, providing sales education programs to individuals and companies. He later founded Cardone Capital, a real estate investment firm focused on multifamily apartment properties across the United States. He authored business books including *The 10X Rule*, *Sell or Be Sold*, and *If You're Not First, You're Last*, which became widely distributed in sales and entrepreneurship circles. He also launched the 10X Growth

Conference, a recurring business event featuring entrepreneurs, investors, and speakers. He has remained active in real estate investment, publishing, and business media into the 2020s.

Gregory Gourdet is a chef, restaurateur who became widely known as a finalist on *Top Chef* and as executive chef of Departure restaurant in Portland, Oregon. After graduating from the Culinary Institute of America, he worked in Jean-Georges Vongerichten's restaurants and later became culinary director of Departure. He authored the cookbook *Everyone's Table* (2021), which won the James Beard Award for Best General Cookbook. In 2022 he opened Kann, a Haitian-inspired restaurant in Portland that won the James Beard Award for Best New Restaurant in 2023. He later received the James Beard Award for Best Chef: Northwest and Pacific. He has also appeared as a television judge and continued expanding his restaurant and media work into the 2020s.

Harry Kane is a soccer player who established his career at Tottenham Hotspur, becoming the club's all-time leading scorer with 280 goals in competitive matches. He won three Premier League Golden Boot awards and, in 2018, became England's all-time leading scorer, later extending his record beyond 70 international goals. As captain, he led England to the 2018 FIFA World Cup semi-finals and the UEFA Euro 2020 final. In 2023 he transferred to Bayern Munich, where he helped the club win the Bundesliga title and continued scoring at a high rate in domestic and European competitions. He has remained one of the leading goal scorers in international and club soccer into the mid-2020s.

Hayley Gibson is a bass player, educator who built her career teaching bass guitar and contemporary music in Australia after completing formal studies in music and education. She taught in schools, polytechnics, and private lessons before founding LearnBass, an online bass instruction platform for adult learners. She developed structured programs including Music for Life, combining technical instruction with goal-based learning and performance preparation. Through workshops, coaching cohorts, and online courses, she expanded her work to support adult musicians returning to playing. She has remained active as a performer, instructor, and program creator, focusing on music education and online training for bass players.

Holly Whitaker is a writer, entrepreneur who gained recognition after launching the blog Hip Sobriety in 2012, which later expanded into digital programs and community-based support initiatives. She founded Tempest, an online platform offering structured courses and peer support. In 2019 she published *Quit Like a Woman*, which became a New York Times bestseller and expanded her readership. She later stepped away from Tempest and continued writing essays, newsletters, and audio projects focused on cultural and behavioral topics. She has remained active as an author and independent media creator into the 2020s.

Jack Harlow is a rapper, actor who first entered the public spotlight after signing with Generation Now and Atlantic Records in 2018 following independent mixtape releases. His single "Whats Poppin" (2020) reached No. 2 on the Billboard Hot 100 and earned a Grammy nomination. His debut studio album *That's What They All Say* (2020) entered the Billboard 200 top ten, and his second album *Come Home the Kids Miss You* (2022) debuted at No. 3, led by the single "First Class," which reached No. 1 on the Billboard Hot 100. He made his acting debut starring in the 2023 film *White Men Can't Jump* and later released his third studio album *Jackman.* (2023).

Jackie Robinson is a baseball player who became the first Black athlete in the modern major leagues when he debuted for the Brooklyn Dodgers in 1947. He won Rookie of the Year that season and was named National League Most Valuable Player in 1949 after leading the league in batting average and stolen bases. Over ten seasons with Brooklyn, he helped the Dodgers win the 1955 World Series and finished with a .311 career batting average. After retiring in 1956, he worked as a business executive, newspaper columnist, and civil rights advocate, including leadership roles with the NAACP. He was inducted into the Baseball Hall of Fame in 1962, and Major League Baseball later retired his uniform number 42 across all teams.

Jada Pinkett Smith is an actor, producer who gained early recognition on the television series *A Different World* beginning in 1991. She later appeared in films including *Menace II Society* (1993) and *Set It Off* (1996), and joined major franchises as Niobe in *The Matrix Reloaded* (2003), *The Matrix Revolutions* (2003), and *The Matrix Resurrections* (2021), and as the voice of Gloria in the *Madagascar* film series. She starred in the television drama *Hawthorne* (2009–2011) and appeared on *Gotham*. In 2018 she co-created and hosted the talk show *Red Table Talk*. She published the memoir *Worthy* in 2023 and has remained active in film, television, and media production.

Jake Paul is a boxer, media personality who entered the public spotlight through videos on Vine and YouTube before transitioning into professional boxing in 2020. He won early bouts against opponents including Nate Robinson, Ben Askren, Tyron Woodley, and Anderson Silva, and headlined major pay-per-view events. In 2021 he co-founded Most Valuable Promotions, which signed boxer Amanda Serrano and promoted major fight cards. He later expanded his career into boxing promotion and sports media, helping produce events distributed on major streaming platforms. He has remained active as both a professional boxer and promoter, contributing to high-profile fights and expanding his presence in sports and entertainment.

James Hetfield is a singer, guitarist who co-founded the band Metallica in 1981 and became its lead vocalist, rhythm guitarist, and primary songwriter. He helped create albums including *Kill 'Em All* (1983), *Ride the Lightning* (1984), *Master of Puppets* (1986), *...And Justice for All* (1988), and *Metallica* (1991), which achieved major commercial success. He continued recording with Metallica on later releases including *St. Anger* (2003), *Death Magnetic* (2008), *Hardwired... to Self-Destruct* (2016), and *72 Seasons* (2023). Metallica won multiple Grammy Awards and was inducted into the Rock and Roll Hall of Fame in 2009. He has remained the band's frontman and a central figure in its global touring and recording career.

James Taylor is a singer, songwriter who gained national recognition with his album *Sweet Baby James* (1970), which included the hit single "Fire and Rain." He followed with *Mud Slide Slim and the Blue Horizon*

(1971), featuring his Grammy-winning recording of "You've Got a Friend." His compilation *Greatest Hits* (1976) became one of the best-selling albums in the United States. Over his career he released more than 20 albums, won multiple Grammy Awards, and earned widespread commercial success. In 2000 he was inducted into both the Rock and Roll Hall of Fame and the Songwriters Hall of Fame. His album *Before This World* (2015) became his first No. 1 on the Billboard 200.

Jamie Campbell Bower is an actor, musician who entered film acting with *Sweeney Todd: The Demon Barber of Fleet Street* (2007). He later appeared as Caius in *The Twilight Saga* film series and portrayed young Gellert Grindelwald in *Harry Potter and the Deathly Hallows – Part 1* (2010) and *Fantastic Beasts: The Crimes of Grindelwald* (2018). He starred as King Arthur in the television series *Camelot* (2011) and played Jace Wayland in *The Mortal Instruments: City of Bones* (2013). In 2022 he gained renewed recognition for portraying Vecna/Henry Creel/001 in *Stranger Things*. He has also worked as a musician, fronting the band Counterfeit and releasing solo material alongside his acting career.

Jamie Lee Curtis is an actor, author who first gained widespread recognition portraying Laurie Strode in *Halloween* (1978), a role she reprised in multiple sequels including the 2018–2022 trilogy. She appeared in films including *Trading Places* (1983), *A Fish Called Wanda* (1988), and *True Lies* (1994), winning a Golden Globe Award for the latter. She later starred in *Freaky Friday* (2003) and appeared in *Knives Out* (2019). She won the Academy Award and Screen Actors Guild Award for Best Supporting Actress for *Everything Everywhere All at Once* (2022). She also appeared in the television series *The Bear*, earning Primetime Emmy Award recognition.

Janeane Garofalo is a comedian, actor who gained national recognition performing stand-up and joining *The Ben Stiller Show* in the early 1990s. She became widely known as Paula on *The Larry Sanders Show*, earning Emmy Award nominations, and later joined the cast of *Saturday Night Live* for the 1994–1995 season. She appeared in films including *Reality Bites* (1994), *The Truth About Cats & Dogs*

(1996), *Romy and Michele's High School Reunion* (1997), and *Wet Hot American Summer* (2001). She voiced Colette in *Ratatouille* (2007) and appeared in television series including *24*, *The West Wing*, and *Criminal Minds*. She has continued performing stand-up comedy and acting in television and film.

Jason Biggs is an actor who became widely known portraying Jim Levenstein in *American Pie* (1999), a role he reprised in sequels including *American Pie 2* (2001), *American Wedding* (2003), and *American Reunion* (2012). He had earlier appeared on the daytime series *As the World Turns*, earning a Daytime Emmy Award nomination. He starred in films including *Loser* (2000), *Saving Silverman* (2001), and *Anything Else* (2003), and appeared in projects such as *Jersey Girl* (2004). He later starred as Larry Bloom on the Netflix series *Orange Is the New Black* (2013–2019) and appeared in television shows including *Mad Love* and *Outmatched*. He has continued working in film, television, and voice acting.

Jason Isbell is a singer, songwriter who entered the public spotlight as a member of Drive-By Truckers from 2001 to 2007 before launching a solo career with *Sirens of the Ditch* (2007). He formed Jason Isbell and the 400 Unit, releasing albums including *Jason Isbell and the 400 Unit* (2009) and *Here We Rest* (2011). His album *Southeastern* (2013) marked a major career milestone and included "Cover Me Up," which won Song of the Year at the Americana Music Honors & Awards. He later released *Something More Than Free* (2015), *The Nashville Sound* (2017), and *Weathervanes* (2023), winning multiple Grammy Awards. He has remained active as a recording artist and touring performer in roots and Americana music.

Jay Shetty is an author, podcast host who gained recognition after creating digital videos on mindfulness and personal development following his time as a monk. He began producing content with HuffPost and later independently, building a large global online audience. In 2019 he launched the podcast *On Purpose*, which became one of the most widely distributed health and wellness podcasts. He authored *Think Like a Monk* (2020) and *8 Rules of Love* (2023), both of which became bestselling books. He also worked in media partnerships and served as Chief Purpose Officer at Calm, contributing to meditation and wellness initiatives. He has remained active in publishing, podcasting, and digital media.

Jennifer Hudson is a singer, actor who became widely known as a finalist on *American Idol* in 2004 before winning the Academy Award for Best Supporting Actress for her film debut in *Dreamgirls* (2006). She released her debut album *Jennifer Hudson* (2008), which won a Grammy Award, and later appeared in films including *The Secret Life of Bees* (2008) and *Respect* (2021), portraying Aretha Franklin. She starred in the Broadway revival of *The Color Purple* and served as a producer on *A Strange Loop*, which contributed to her achieving EGOT status. In 2022 she launched the syndicated daytime program *The Jennifer Hudson Show*, expanding her career into television hosting.

Jermain Defoe is a soccer player who gained early recognition as a prolific scorer in the English Premier League with clubs including West Ham United, Tottenham Hotspur, Portsmouth, and Sunderland. He made nearly 500 Premier League appearances and scored more than 160 goals, placing him among the league's top scorers. He earned 57 caps for England between 2004 and 2017, scoring 20 international goals and appearing in the 2010 FIFA World Cup. He later played for Rangers, helping the club win the Scottish Premiership title in the 2020–2021 season. After retiring from professional soccer, he became involved in coaching and charitable work, including founding the Jermain Defoe Foundation.

Jessica Simpson is a singer, entrepreneur who entered the public spotlight with her debut album *Sweet Kisses* (1999), which included the hit single "I Wanna Love You Forever." She released subsequent albums including *In This Skin* (2003) and starred in the MTV reality series *Newlyweds: Nick & Jessica* (2003–2005). She later appeared in films including *The Dukes of Hazzard* (2005). She founded the Jessica Simpson Collection, a fashion and lifestyle brand that expanded into apparel, footwear, and accessories through major retail partnerships. In 2021 she regained full ownership of the company. She has also authored bestselling books and remained active in business and media.

Jessie J is a singer, songwriter who gained international recognition with her debut single "Do It Like a Dude" (2010) and her breakthrough hit "Price Tag" (2011). Her debut album *Who You Are* (2011) produced multiple U.K. top-ten singles and established her global pop career. She later released albums including *Alive* (2013) and *Sweet Talker* (2014), featuring the single "Bang Bang" with Ariana Grande and Nicki Minaj, which reached No. 3 on the Billboard Hot 100. In 2018 she won the Chinese television competition *Singer*, becoming the first international artist to win the program. She has continued recording, touring, and releasing new music into the 2020s.

Jim Carrey is an actor, comedian who became widely known after starring in three 1994 film comedies: *Ace Ventura: Pet Detective*, *The Mask*, and *Dumb and Dumber*. He followed with *Batman Forever* (1995) and *Ace Ventura: When Nature Calls* (1995), then shifted into dramatic and character roles in *The Truman Show* (1998), *Man on the Moon* (1999), and *Eternal Sunshine of the Spotless Mind* (2004), winning two Golden Globe Awards for the first two. He later headlined films including *How the Grinch Stole Christmas* (2000) and *Bruce Almighty* (2003), and played Dr. Robotnik in the *Sonic the Hedgehog* film series (2020–2024).

Jimmy Connors is a tennis player who became famous in the 1970s as a dominant figure in men's tennis, winning 109 Open Era singles titles and eight major singles championships. He won five US Opens (on three different surfaces), two Wimbledons, and one Australian Open, and reached world No. 1 in 1974. He held the top ranking for 160 consecutive weeks and 268 total weeks, and finished as the year-end No. 1 from 1974 through 1978. In 1991, at age 39, he reached the US Open semifinals as a wildcard. After retiring, he worked in tennis media and coached, including a stint with Andy Roddick.

Jocko Willink is a retired U.S. Navy SEAL officer who served 20 years in the Navy, including leadership of SEAL Team 3's Task Unit Bruiser during the Iraq War Battle of Ramadi. His unit received multiple commendations, and he was awarded the Silver Star and Bronze Star with Combat "V." After combat deployments, he served as officer in charge of training for West Coast SEAL Teams. He retired in 2010 and co-founded the leadership consulting firm Echelon Front. He launched the Jocko Podcast in 2015 and co-authored Extreme Ownership and subsequent books. He has also operated businesses including Origin USA and Jocko Fuel, extending his leadership teachings into publishing, training, and consumer products.

Joe Biden is a politician who served as the 46th president of the United States from 2021 to 2025 after nearly five decades in federal office. First elected U.S. senator from Delaware in 1972, he served six terms, chaired the Senate Judiciary and Foreign Relations Committees, and helped pass the Violence Against Women Act. He was vice president under Barack Obama from 2009 to 2017, participating in economic recovery efforts and passage of the Affordable Care Act. Elected president in 2020, he signed the American Rescue Plan, Infrastructure Investment and Jobs Act, and CHIPS and Science Act, and oversaw the U.S. withdrawal from Afghanistan in 2021. His administration supported Ukraine following Russia's 2022 invasion and approved Finland and Sweden's accession to NATO.

Joe Namath is a former professional football quarterback who became widely known after leading the New York Jets to victory in Super Bowl III in January 1969, guaranteeing a win over the Baltimore Colts. He joined the Jets in 1965 after starring at the University of Alabama and was named AFL MVP in 1968. In 1967 he became the first professional quarterback to pass for more than 4,000 yards in a season. Over 13 seasons with the Jets and Los Angeles Rams, he threw for 27,663 yards and 173 touchdowns, earned five Pro Bowl selections, and led his league in passing yards three times. His Super Bowl III victory helped legitimize the AFL ahead of the AFL–NFL merger, and he was inducted into the Pro Football Hall of Fame in 1985.

Joe Rogan is a stand-up comedian, podcast host, and UFC commentator who entered the public spotlight in the 1990s with roles on sitcoms including NewsRadio. He hosted NBC's Fear Factor from 2001 to 2006 and its 2011 revival, expanding his national television presence. A martial artist with competition experience in taekwondo, he began working with the UFC in 1997 and became a longtime color commentator, earning multiple World MMA Awards. In 2009 he launched The Joe Rogan Experience, an interview podcast that became one of the most widely distributed shows globally. In 2020 he signed an exclusive licensing agreement with Spotify, and in 2024 reached a new multi-year distribution deal allowing the show to expand across additional platforms while maintaining Spotify partnership.

Joe Walsh is a guitarist, singer, and songwriter who gained national recognition in the late 1960s as a member of the James Gang, contributing to hits including Funk #49 and Walk Away and several gold-certified albums. After leaving the band in 1972, he formed Barnstorm and launched a solo career with recordings including Rocky Mountain Way and multiple charting albums. In 1975 he joined the Eagles, contributing guitar, vocals, and songwriting to Hotel California (1976) and later releases including The Long Run (1979). He also maintained solo work, released additional albums, and toured extensively. Walsh was inducted into the Rock and Roll Hall of Fame with the Eagles in 1998 and has continued performing with the band and as a solo artist into the 2020s.

John Goodman is an actor who entered the public spotlight on television as Dan Conner on the sitcom *Roseanne*, beginning in 1988, earning a Golden Globe Award in 1993 and multiple Emmy nominations, and later reprising the role in *The Conners*. He built a parallel film career with roles in Coen brothers projects including *Raising Arizona* (1987), *Barton Fink* (1991), *The Big Lebowski* (1998), and *O Brother, Where Art Thou?* (2000). He voiced Sulley in Pixar's *Monsters, Inc.* (2001) and its sequel and prequel. His later film work included *Argo* (2012) and *10 Cloverfield Lane* (2016), and he appeared in HBO's *Treme* (2010–2013). He received a star on the Hollywood Walk of Fame in 2017 and has continued acting in television and film into the 2020s.

John Mayer is a guitarist, singer, and songwriter who gained national recognition with his debut major-label album *Room for Squares* (2001), which produced "No Such Thing" and "Your Body Is a Wonderland," the latter winning the 2003 Grammy Award for Best Male Pop Vocal Performance. His follow-up album *Heavier Things*

(2003) debuted at No. 1 on the Billboard 200 and included "Daughters," which won Song of the Year at the 2005 Grammys. He expanded into blues with the John Mayer Trio and released *Continuum* (2006), which won Best Pop Vocal Album. Later albums include *Born and Raised* (2012), *The Search for Everything* (2017), and *Sob Rock* (2021). He has won seven Grammy Awards, sold millions of records worldwide, and since 2015 has performed as a guitarist and vocalist with Dead & Company.

John Mulaney is a stand-up comedian, writer, and actor who emerged as a leading figure as a writer on *Saturday Night Live* beginning in 2008, where he co-created the Stefon character and won Primetime Emmy Awards for Outstanding Writing for a Variety Series. He released stand-up specials including *The Top Part* (2009), *New in Town* (2012), *The Comeback Kid* (2015), *Kid Gorgeous at Radio City* (2018), and *Baby J* (2023), with *Kid Gorgeous* and *Baby J* winning Emmy Awards for Outstanding Writing for a Variety Special. He created and starred in the sitcom *Mulaney* (2014–2015), co-wrote and performed *Oh, Hello* on Broadway, voiced Spider-Ham in *Spider-Man: Into the Spider-Verse* (2018), and has hosted *Saturday Night Live* multiple times, joining the Five-Timers Club in 2022.

John Wooden is a college basketball coach who became head coach at UCLA in 1948 and built one of the most successful programs in NCAA history. His teams won 10 NCAA championships between 1964 and 1975, including seven consecutive titles from 1967 to 1973, and completed four undefeated seasons. UCLA also set an NCAA men's basketball record with 88 consecutive victories from 1971 to 1974 and won 38 straight NCAA tournament games during its championship run. Wooden compiled a 620–147 record at UCLA before retiring in 1975. He was inducted into the Naismith Memorial Basketball Hall of Fame as a player in 1960 and as a coach in 1973, and his "Pyramid of Success" became widely used in coaching, education, and leadership training.

Johnny Manziel is a former American football quarterback who gained national recognition at Texas A&M, where he became the first freshman to win the Heisman Trophy in 2012. That season he set an SEC single-season record with 5,116 total yards, including 3,706 passing and 1,410 rushing, and led Texas A&M to an 11–2 record and a win over top-ranked Alabama. He entered the NFL as the 22nd overall pick in the 2014 draft by the Cleveland Browns, appearing in 14 games and making eight starts across two seasons. After leaving the NFL in 2016, he played professionally for the Hamilton Tiger-Cats and Montreal Alouettes in the CFL and later appeared in the Alliance of American Football and Fan Controlled Football.

Jordan Peterson is a Canadian clinical psychologist, author, and professor who became widely known after his academic work at the University of Toronto and public lectures on psychology, culture, and belief. After earning a PhD from McGill University, he taught at Harvard University from 1993 to 1998 before joining the University of Toronto, where he became a full professor. He published the scholarly book *Maps of Meaning* (1999) and later reached a mass audience with *12 Rules for Life* (2018) and *Beyond Order* (2021), which together sold millions of copies worldwide. His lectures and interviews accumulated hundreds of millions of views online, and he launched *The Jordan Peterson Podcast* and self-authoring programs. In 2024 he was appointed chancellor of Ralston College, expanding his role in independent higher education.

Josh Hamilton is a former baseball player who rose to prominence with the Texas Rangers after debuting in Major League Baseball with the Cincinnati Reds in 2007. He joined Texas in 2008 and became a five-time All-Star, winning the American League MVP Award in 2010 after batting .359 with 32 home runs and a league-leading 1.044 OPS. He helped lead the Rangers to consecutive World Series appearances in 2010 and 2011 and earned ALCS MVP honors in 2010. Hamilton later played for the Los Angeles Angels and returned briefly to Texas before his final MLB season in 2015. Across his career he hit 200 home runs and won three Silver Slugger Awards, finishing as one of the most productive hitters of his era.

Josh Peck is an actor and digital creator who first emerged as a leading figure as a cast member on Nickelodeon's *The Amanda Show* (2000–2002) before starring as Josh Nichols on *Drake & Josh* (2004–2007). He voiced Eddie in multiple *Ice Age* animated films and appeared in movies including *Mean Creek* (2004) and *The Wackness* (2008). He later starred in television series such as *Grandfathered* (2015–2016) and Disney+'s *Turner & Hooch* (2021), and had a recurring role on *How I Met Your Father* (2022–2023). He launched a YouTube channel in 2017, building a large digital audience, and published the memoir *Happy People Are Annoying* (2022), expanding his work into writing and podcasting alongside his screen career.

Julien Baker is a singer-songwriter who achieved early recognition with the release of her debut album *Sprained Ankle* (2015) while a student at Middle Tennessee State University. The album drew critical attention and led to wider distribution and touring. She followed with *Turn Out the Lights* (2017), which expanded her audience, and *Little Oblivions* (2021), her first album to enter the Billboard 200 top 40. In parallel, she co-founded the indie rock trio boygenius with Phoebe Bridgers and Lucy Dacus; their debut studio album *The Record* (2023) reached the Billboard 200 top 10 and won multiple Grammy Awards. Alongside solo and group releases, she has performed internationally and contributed to collaborative projects across the indie rock genre.

Karlyn Pipes is a swimmer and coach who established one of the most extensive records in Masters swimming after returning to competition in her early 30s. She quickly set a Masters world record in the 200-meter backstroke and went on to rank first in the United States in multiple events. Over subsequent decades she set more than 200 FINA Masters world records and over 300 U.S. Masters national records across freestyle, backstroke, breaststroke, and butterfly in multiple age groups. She earned repeated World Masters Swimmer of the Year honors and was inducted into the International Swimming Hall of Fame. She later authored the memoir *The Do-Over* and developed a career as a swim technique coach, author, and speaker.

Kat Von D (Katherine von Drachenberg) is a tattoo artist, television personality, entrepreneur who rose to prominence after appearing on TLC's *Miami Ink* in 2005 and then leading the spin-off series *LA Ink* (2007–2011). She operated the West Hollywood shop High Voltage Tattoo during her TV rise and set a Guinness World Records mark by tattooing 400 people in 24 hours. In 2008 she launched Kat Von D

Beauty, a cosmetics brand that expanded internationally; she later sold her ownership stake and fully exited the business, which continued under the KVD branding. She has also released books, music projects, and a vegan footwear line, extending her work beyond tattooing into publishing and consumer products.

Kate Moss is a model who gained international recognition in the early 1990s through appearances in *The Face* and advertising campaigns for Calvin Klein, including its Obsession fragrance and jeans campaigns. She became one of the most in-demand fashion models of her era, appearing on hundreds of magazine covers and fronting campaigns for brands including Chanel, Gucci, Versace, Burberry, and Rimmel. She maintained a continuous presence in runway, editorial, and advertising work across multiple decades. In 2016 she founded the Kate Moss Agency, representing models and creative talent, and later launched the Cosmoss wellness and lifestyle brand. She has also collaborated on fashion collections and fragrances, extending her work into design, talent management, and brand development.

Kathryn Helgaas Burgum is a public official and advocate who became First Lady of North Dakota in 2016 when Doug Burgum assumed the governorship. She helped lead the state's Recovery Reinvented initiative, launched in 2017 to address substance use through education, prevention, and community engagement. She chairs the advisory council supporting the program and has helped organize annual Recovery Reinvented conferences attended by participants across the United States. Her work has included promoting public awareness campaigns, supporting expanded access to naloxone, and collaborating with state and national organizations on public health initiatives. In 2024 she received the Pioneer Award at the eighth Recovery Reinvented event, recognizing her leadership in advancing statewide and national efforts related to substance use awareness and policy.

Kathy Griffin is a stand-up comedian, actor, and television personality who became widely known after creating and starring in the Bravo reality series *Kathy Griffin: My Life on the D-List* (2005–2010). The show ran six seasons, earned multiple Emmy nominations, and won two Primetime Emmy Awards for Outstanding Reality Program. She released more than 20 televised stand-up specials, earning a Guinness World Records recognition, and won the Grammy Award for Best Comedy Album in 2014 for *Calm Down Gurrl*. She has also appeared in television series including *Suddenly Susan* and published bestselling memoirs. After 2020 she returned to live touring, digital content, and media appearances, continuing her career across stand-up, television, and publishing.

Keith Urban is a country singer, songwriter, and guitarist who established his solo career in the United States with his self-titled album *Keith Urban* (1999) and his first No. 1 country single, "But for the Grace of God." He followed with albums including *Golden Road* (2002), which produced "Somebody Like You," later named Billboard's top country song of the 2000s decade. He has released more than a dozen studio albums and scored over 20 No. 1 singles on the Billboard Hot Country Songs chart, including "Blue Ain't Your Color" and "Wasted Time." He has won four Grammy Awards and was inducted into the Grand Ole Opry in 2012. He also served as a judge on *American Idol* and has continued touring and releasing new music into the 2020s.

Kelly Osbourne is a television personality, singer, and presenter who became widely known after appearing on MTV's reality series *The Osbournes* (2002–2005), which won the Primetime Emmy Award for Outstanding Reality Program. She released two studio albums, *Shut Up* (2002) and *Sleeping in the Nothing* (2005), and reached the finals of *Dancing with the Stars* in 2009. She later cohosted E!'s *Fashion Police* from 2010 to 2015 and served as a red-carpet correspondent and fashion commentator. She also voiced Hildy Gloom in Disney XD's *The 7D* and appeared as a judge on *Project Runway Junior* and *Australia's Got Talent*. She has continued working in television, fashion media, and entertainment presenting.

Kelly Ripa is an actor, producer, and television host who gained national recognition playing Hayley Vaughan on *All My Children* from 1990 to 2002. In 2001 she became cohost of the syndicated morning talk show *Live!* alongside Regis Philbin, later leading versions including *Live with Kelly and Mark*. She has hosted the program for more than two decades, helping it remain a consistent presence in daytime television ratings. She has won multiple Daytime Emmy Awards for Outstanding Entertainment Talk Show Host and was named a Disney Legend in 2024. In addition to hosting, she has acted in television projects and co-founded Milojo Productions with Mark Consuelos, producing television and film content.

Kevin Kreider is a model, actor, and television personality who gained widespread visibility as a cast member on Netflix's *Bling Empire*, which premiered in 2021. He previously worked as a fitness model and commercial actor, including campaigns for brands such as Abercrombie & Fitch and Gillette, and spoke publicly on identity and representation through talks at TEDx and corporate events. He expanded into acting with roles in independent films including *Asian Persuasion* and appeared in reality competition series such as *The Traitors*. He later co-founded ALLS Productions to develop film and television projects focused on Asian-led stories and launched the beverage brand SANS by Taejin, extending his work into entrepreneurship alongside modeling and screen roles.

Khabib Nurmagomedov is a mixed martial artist who achieved global recognition after joining the UFC in 2012 and compiling an undefeated professional record of 29–0. He won the vacant UFC lightweight championship at UFC 223 in April 2018 and successfully defended the title three times, including a high-profile bout against Conor McGregor at UFC 229, one of the highest-selling pay-per-view events in MMA history. Known for his grappling and takedown-focused style, he set a UFC record with 21 takedowns in a single fight. He retired from competition in 2020 as the undefeated UFC lightweight champion and was inducted into the UFC Hall of Fame in 2022. After retiring, he transitioned into coaching and promoting mixed martial arts.

Kit Harington is an actor who gained international recognition after being cast as Jon Snow in HBO's *Game of Thrones*, appearing in all eight seasons from 2011 to 2019. His performance earned a Primetime Emmy Award nomination and helped establish the series as one of television's most widely viewed dramas. He previously originated the role of Albert Narracott in the West End production of *War Horse*.

During and after *Game of Thrones*, he appeared in films including *Pompeii* (2014) and *Testament of Youth* (2014), voiced Eret in the *How to Train Your Dragon* franchise, and joined the Marvel Cinematic Universe as Dane Whitman in *Eternals* (2021). He later returned to stage and television roles, continuing his acting career across multiple platforms.

Kris Kristofferson is a songwriter, singer, and actor who became a central figure in country music after writing hit songs recorded by major artists in the late 1960s and early 1970s. His compositions include "Me and Bobby McGee," "For the Good Times," "Sunday Mornin' Comin' Down," and "Help Me Make It Through the Night," with the latter two earning major country and Grammy honors. He launched a recording career with albums such as *Kristofferson* (1970) and scored a No. 1 country hit with "Why Me." He later joined Johnny Cash, Waylon Jennings, and Willie Nelson in the group the Highwaymen. As an actor, he starred in *A Star Is Born* (1976), winning a Golden Globe Award. He was inducted into the Country Music Hall of Fame in 2004 and received a Grammy Lifetime Achievement Award in 2014.

Kristin Davis is an actor and producer who gained global recognition portraying Charlotte York on HBO's *Sex and the City* from 1998 to 2004. She earned Primetime Emmy and Golden Globe nominations for the role and reprised the character in two feature films released in 2008 and 2010, as well as the sequel series *And Just Like That…*. She previously appeared in television series including *Melrose Place* and has worked in television films, voice acting, and producing. Beyond acting, she partnered with the Sheldrick Wildlife Trust beginning in 2009, supporting elephant conservation and executive-producing the documentary *Gardeners of Eden* (2014). Her work has included producing and starring in film and television projects while contributing to wildlife conservation advocacy.

Kyle Richards is an actor, television personality, producer, and entrepreneur who gained early recognition as Lindsey Wallace in *Halloween* (1978) and as a child actor on *Little House on the Prairie*. She appeared in numerous television and film roles before joining *The*

Real Housewives of Beverly Hills in 2010 as an original cast member, remaining one of the franchise's longest-tenured participants. She reprised her *Halloween* role in *Halloween Kills* (2021) and *Halloween Ends* (2022). Richards co-executive-produced the Paramount Network series *American Woman* (2018), inspired by her upbringing. She also launched fashion and retail ventures, including the Kyle x Shahida clothing line, and has remained active in television production, acting, and brand collaborations into the 2020s.

Lamar Odom is a former professional basketball player who became widely known as a versatile forward with the Los Angeles Lakers during their late-2000s championship runs. Drafted fourth overall by the Los Angeles Clippers in 1999, he played 14 NBA seasons, averaging 13.3 points, 8.4 rebounds, and 3.7 assists across 961 games. He won two NBA championships with the Lakers in 2009 and 2010 and received the NBA Sixth Man of the Year Award in 2011. He also appeared on the reality television series *Khloé & Lamar* (2011–2012). After retiring from basketball, he participated in media projects, celebrity boxing exhibitions, and business ventures, including wellness-related partnerships and brand licensing initiatives launched in the 2020s.

Lana Del Rey (Elizabeth Grant) is a singer-songwriter who rose to prominence with the viral single "Video Games" (2011) and her major-label debut *Born to Die* (2012). The album achieved multi-platinum certifications worldwide and became one of the longest-charting albums on the Billboard 200, remaining on the chart for over 500 weeks. She followed with albums including *Ultraviolence* (2014), *Honeymoon* (2015), *Norman F**ing Rockwell!** (2019), *Chemtrails over the Country Club* (2021), *Did You Know That There's a Tunnel Under Ocean Blvd* (2023), and *Lasso* (2024). She has received multiple Grammy nominations and won awards including a Brit Award and Billboard honors. Her collaborations include charting singles with The Weeknd and Taylor Swift, sustaining international chart and touring presence into the 2020s.

Lane Kiffin is a football coach who became the NFL's youngest modern head coach with the Oakland Raiders in 2007 at age 31. After assistant roles at USC, he led Tennessee in 2009 and USC from 2010 to 2013, then served as offensive coordinator at Alabama from 2014 to 2016, helping the program win the 2015 national championship. As head coach at Florida Atlantic from 2017 to 2019, he won two Conference USA titles and an 11–3 debut season. He became head coach at Ole Miss in 2020, producing multiple double-digit-win seasons, including an 11–2 season in 2023 capped by a Peach Bowl victory. His tenure included several top-10 finishes and established the program among the SEC's consistent contenders into the mid-2020s.

Larry Ellison is an entrepreneur and technologist who co-founded Software Development Laboratories in 1977, later renamed Oracle Corporation, to commercialize relational database software. After early contracts with government and corporate clients, Oracle went public in 1986 and recovered from financial setbacks to become a leading enterprise database vendor with Oracle7 in 1992. As CEO from 1977 to 2014, he led acquisitions including PeopleSoft, Siebel Systems, Hyperion, and Sun Microsystems, expanding Oracle into applications, hardware, and enterprise systems. After stepping down as CEO, he remained executive chairman and chief technology officer, directing Oracle's expansion into cloud computing and AI infrastructure. He also acquired most of the Hawaiian island of Lanai and became one of the world's wealthiest individuals through his Oracle holdings.

Laura McKowen is an author, podcaster, and entrepreneur who transitioned from advertising into writing and media, gaining recognition with her memoir *We Are the Luckiest* (2020). After building an audience through blogging and cohosting the podcast *HOME*, she expanded her platform through books, speaking, and digital programming. Her second book, *Push Off From Here* (2023), further developed her themes of personal change and emotional resilience. In 2020 she founded The Luckiest Club, an online membership community offering structured meetings, workshops, and peer support. She has contributed essays and commentary to national publications and appeared on major broadcast programs. Through writing, podcasting, and leadership of her digital platform, she established a sustained career in publishing and online community development.

Leslie Jamison is a novelist, essayist, and critic who gained recognition with her essay collection *The Empathy Exams* (2014), which became a New York Times bestseller and won the Graywolf Press Nonfiction Prize. Her debut novel *The Gin Closet* appeared in 2010, followed by *The Recovering* (2018), a nonfiction work blending memoir, literary criticism, and cultural analysis. She expanded her nonfiction with *Make It Scream, Make It Burn* (2019) and the memoir *Splinters* (2024). In addition to her books, she has published essays and criticism in major literary and national publications. She has also taught creative writing and directed the nonfiction concentration at Columbia University's School of the Arts, contributing to contemporary literary nonfiction through both writing and academic leadership.

Lewis Hamilton is a Formula 1 driver who debuted with McLaren in 2007 and won his first World Drivers' Championship in 2008. After moving to Mercedes in 2013, he secured six additional titles between 2014 and 2020, tying Michael Schumacher's record of seven championships. He became the first driver to surpass 100 race wins and 100 pole positions and accumulated more than 200 podium finishes and over 5,000 career points. He drove for Mercedes through the 2024 season before joining Ferrari for the 2025 Formula 1 season, marking a major team change after more than a decade. Across nearly two decades in Formula 1, he has remained among the sport's most statistically successful drivers by wins, poles, and championships.

Lily Allen is a singer-songwriter and actor who gained international recognition with her debut album *Alright, Still* (2006), which sold over 2 million copies and earned a Grammy nomination. Her second album *It's Not Me, It's You* (2009) debuted at No. 1 in the U.K. and Australia and produced the Brit Award-winning single "The Fear." She later released *Sheezus* (2014), which also reached No. 1 in the U.K., and *No Shame* (2018), which received a Mercury Prize nomination. In theater, she made her West End acting debut in *2:22 A Ghost Story* (2021), earning an Olivier Award nomination for Best Actress. Alongside music, she has pursued acting, publishing, and stage projects while maintaining a recording career.

Lindsay Lohan is an actor and singer who rose to prominence as a child star in Disney's *The Parent Trap* (1998) before leading teen films including *Freaky Friday* (2003) and *Mean Girls* (2004), both major box-office successes. She launched a music career with the platinum album *Speak* (2004) and followed with *A Little More Personal (Raw)* (2005). After reduced film output in the late 2000s and 2010s, she returned to acting with Netflix releases including *Falling for Christmas* (2022) and *Irish Wish* (2024). She expanded her comeback with additional film and streaming projects while maintaining credits across film, television, and music spanning more than three decades.

Lisa Riley is an actor and television presenter who gained national recognition after joining *Emmerdale* as Mandy Dingle in 1995, winning the 1996 National Television Award for Most Popular Newcomer and returning as a regular from 2019. She hosted ITV's *You've Been Framed!* from 1998 to 2002, drawing audiences above 10 million and becoming one of the network's youngest prime-time presenters. She appeared in television dramas including *Fat Friends*, *Waterloo Road*, and *Three Girls*, and reached the semi-finals of *Strictly Come Dancing* in 2012. She also built a stage career in touring productions and pantomime while continuing regular television appearances across drama and entertainment formats into the 2020s.

Logan Paul is a digital creator, professional wrestler, boxer, and entrepreneur who built a large online audience through Vine and YouTube, where his Logan Paul Vlogs channel surpassed 23 million subscribers. He ranked among Forbes' highest-paid YouTube creators in 2017 and 2018 and later headlined boxing events against KSI in 2018 and 2019 and an exhibition with Floyd Mayweather in 2021. In WWE, he debuted at WrestleMania 38 in 2022, became a regular performer, and won the WWE United States Championship in November 2023. As co-founder of Prime Hydration, launched in 2022 with KSI, he helped scale the beverage brand to over $1 billion in annual retail sales and global distribution across major markets.

Lucy Hale is an actor and singer who rose to prominence starring as Aria Montgomery on *Pretty Little Liars* (2010–2017), appearing in all 160 episodes and receiving multiple Teen Choice Awards, a People's

Choice Award, and a Gracie Award. She began on television with roles on *Drake & Josh*, *Wizards of Waverly Place*, and *Privileged*, and later led series including *Life Sentence* (2018), *Katy Keene* (2020), and *Ragdoll* (2021). In film, she starred in *Truth or Dare* (2018), *Fantasy Island* (2020), and romantic comedies such as *The Hating Game* (2021) and *Which Brings Me to You* (2023). She released the country album *Road Between* in 2014 and has continued acting in films and television into the mid-2020s.

Macklemore is a rapper and songwriter who gained global recognition after independently releasing *The Heist* (2012) with producer Ryan Lewis, which debuted at No. 2 on the Billboard 200 and produced the No. 1 singles "Thrift Shop" and "Can't Hold Us." The duo won four Grammy Awards in 2014, including Best New Artist and Best Rap Album, becoming one of the most prominent independent acts to achieve mainstream chart success. He followed with *This Unruly Mess I've Made* (2016) and solo albums *Gemini* (2017) and *Ben* (2023), which included charting singles and international touring. His releases have accumulated billions of streams, and he has continued performing and releasing music independently into the mid-2020s.

Mandy Moore is a singer and actor who first gained mainstream attention with her debut single "Candy" (1999) and album *So Real*, which achieved platinum certification in the United States. She released five studio albums by 2009, including *Coverage* (2003) and *Wild Hope* (2007), while transitioning into acting with film roles in *The Princess Diaries* (2001) and *A Walk to Remember* (2002). She voiced Rapunzel in Disney's *Tangled* (2010) and its related projects, expanding her work in animation. From 2016 to 2022 she starred as Rebecca Pearson on NBC's *This Is Us*, earning Golden Globe and Emmy nominations and sharing multiple Screen Actors Guild Awards with the cast. She has continued recording music, acting in television and film, and performing voice roles into the mid-2020s.

Marc Andreessen is a software developer and venture capitalist who co-created the Mosaic web browser in 1993 while at the University of Illinois, helping popularize the graphical internet. In 1994 he co-founded Netscape Communications, whose Navigator browser gained dominant early market share and whose 1995 IPO became a milestone in the dot-com boom; AOL acquired Netscape in 1999 for about $4.2 billion. He later co-founded Loudcloud, renamed Opsware, which Hewlett-Packard acquired in 2007 for $1.6 billion, and launched the social platform Ning. In 2009 he co-founded venture capital firm Andreessen Horowitz, which grew into one of Silicon Valley's largest firms and backed companies including Facebook, Airbnb, Coinbase, Slack, and GitHub. He has remained a general partner guiding investments across software, crypto, and artificial intelligence.

Mark Manson is a writer who gained global recognition after publishing the self-help book *The Subtle Art of Not Giving a F*ck** in 2016, following earlier success with his blog and the independently published book *Models* (2011). *The Subtle Art of Not Giving a F*ck** reached No. 1 on the *New York Times* bestseller list, remained on the list for years, and sold more than 12 million copies worldwide. His follow-up book *Everything Is F*cked: A Book About Hope** (2019) also became a No. 1 *New York Times* bestseller. He co-wrote Will Smith's memoir *Will* (2021), which reached No. 1 on bestseller lists. By the mid-2020s his books had sold millions of copies globally and were translated into dozens of languages, supporting international speaking, courses, and media projects.

Mary J Blige is a singer, songwriter, and actor who rose to prominence after releasing her debut album *What's the 411?* in 1992, which blended R&B vocals with hip-hop production and produced hits including "Real Love." Her second album *My Life* (1994) expanded her audience, and later releases such as *Share My World* (1997), *The Breakthrough* (2005), and *Growing Pains* (2007) debuted at No. 1 on the *Billboard* 200. The single "Family Affair" became her first No. 1 on the *Billboard* Hot 100. She has won nine Grammy Awards and sold more than 50 million albums worldwide. In film, she earned Academy Award nominations for Best Supporting Actress and Best Original Song for *Mudbound* (2017), becoming the first person nominated in both categories in the same year.

Mary Karr is a memoirist, poet, and essayist who gained national recognition with her memoir *The Liars' Club* (1995), which became a

New York Times bestseller and helped expand the contemporary memoir genre. She followed with memoirs *Cherry* (2000) and *Lit* (2009), which continued her autobiographical narrative into adulthood. She has also published several poetry collections, including *Viper Rum* (1998) and *Sinners Welcome* (2006), and her craft guide *The Art of Memoir* (2015) became a bestseller used in writing programs. Her essays and poems have appeared in publications including *The New Yorker* and *The Atlantic*. She has taught at Syracuse University and received fellowships from the Guggenheim Foundation, National Endowment for the Arts, and Radcliffe Institute.

Matthew Perry is an actor who became widely known for portraying Chandler Bing on the NBC sitcom *Friends* from 1994 to 2004, appearing in all 236 episodes as cast salaries reached $1 million per episode and the 2004 finale drew over 52 million U.S. viewers. He also starred in films including *The Whole Nine Yards* (2000) and *17 Again* (2009), and earned Emmy nominations for *Friends* and *The Ron Clark Story* (2006). He later co-created and starred in the sitcom *Mr. Sunshine* (2011) and appeared in *The Odd Couple* (2015–2017). His memoir *Friends, Lovers, and the Big Terrible Thing* (2022) became a bestseller. Perry died on October 28, 2023, and his legacy continued through the Matthew Perry Foundation.

Maxx Crosby is an NFL defensive end who emerged as a central figure in the Las Vegas Raiders' defense after being selected in the fourth round of the 2019 NFL Draft out of Eastern Michigan. He recorded 10 sacks as a rookie and developed into one of the league's most productive edge rushers, earning multiple Pro Bowl selections and first-team All-Pro honors. In 2022 he led the NFL in tackles for loss and was named a team captain. By early 2026 he had accumulated 69.5 career sacks and more than 430 total tackles, placing him among franchise leaders. In 2025 he signed a three-year, $106.5 million contract extension with $91.5 million guaranteed, setting a record for non-quarterbacks at the time.

Mel Gibson is an actor and filmmaker who rose to prominence through Australian films before becoming a global box-office lead and Academy Award–winning director. He gained international recognition starring in the *Mad Max* series (1979–1985) and the *Lethal Weapon* franchise (1987–1998). He directed, produced, and starred in *Braveheart* (1995), which won Academy Awards for Best Picture and Best Director. His subsequent directing projects included *The Passion of the Christ* (2004), which grossed over $600 million worldwide, and *Apocalypto* (2006). He returned to directing with *Hacksaw Ridge* (2016), earning Academy Award nominations for Best Picture and Best Director. He has continued acting in films such as *Blood Father* (2016) and *Dragged Across Concrete* (2018), extending his screen and directing career beyond four decades.

Melanie Griffith is an actor who established her film career in the 1980s and became widely known after starring in major studio and television productions. She gained attention in films including *Body Double* (1984) and *Something Wild* (1986), then received an Academy Award nomination and won a Golden Globe for Best Actress for *Working Girl* (1988). She continued with leading and supporting roles in films such as *Pacific Heights* (1990), *Milk Money* (1994), and *Lolita* (1997). On television she earned Golden Globe and Emmy nominations for *Buffalo Girls* (1995) and an Emmy nomination for *RKO 281* (1999). She later appeared in independent films, television projects, and stage productions, including her Broadway debut in *Chicago* (2003), sustaining a screen and stage career spanning five decades.

Michael Landon is an actor, writer, director, and producer who became a central figure in American television through starring roles and creative control on three long-running network dramas. He gained national recognition as Little Joe Cartwright on *Bonanza* (1959–1973), appearing in more than 400 episodes while also writing and directing. He later created, produced, wrote, directed, and starred in *Little House on the Prairie* (1974–1983), which ran nine seasons and continued through television films. He then led and executive-produced *Highway to Heaven* (1984–1989), appearing in 111 episodes. Across his career he received multiple Emmy nominations and People's Choice Awards and was inducted into the National Cowboy & Western Heritage Museum's Hall of Great Western Performers. He remained active in television production until his death in 1991.

Michael Phelps is a swimmer who became the most decorated Olympian in history through record-setting performances across five Olympic Games. He qualified for his first Olympics at age 15 in Sydney 2000, then won six gold and two bronze medals at Athens 2004. At Beijing 2008 he won eight gold medals, breaking Mark Spitz's record for most golds at a single Olympics. He added four golds and two silvers in London 2012 and five golds and one silver in Rio 2016, finishing with 28 Olympic medals, including 23 gold. He also won 26 World Championship gold medals and set multiple world records in butterfly, individual medley, and relay events. After retiring in 2016, he established the Michael Phelps Foundation to promote swimming instruction and healthy living.

Mike McDaniel is an NFL coach who entered the public spotlight in 2022 when the Miami Dolphins hired him as head coach. He began in the NFL as a Denver Broncos coaching intern in 2005, then held offensive assistant roles with the Houston Texans and Washington Redskins, coached wide receivers for the Cleveland Browns, and served as an offensive assistant with the Atlanta Falcons, reaching Super Bowl LI. He joined the San Francisco 49ers in 2017, working as a run game specialist and run game coordinator before becoming offensive coordinator in 2021 and reaching Super Bowl LIV. McDaniel coached the Dolphins from 2022–2025, posting a 35–33 regular-season record and making the playoffs in 2022 and 2023. He was dismissed after the 2025 season and became the Los Angeles Chargers' offensive coordinator in January 2026.

Miley Cyrus is a singer, songwriter, and actor who became widely known after starring in the Disney Channel series *Hannah Montana* (2006–2011), which generated chart-topping soundtracks, tours, and a theatrical film. She launched a solo recording career with *Meet Miley Cyrus* (2007) and later released albums including *Bangerz* (2013), *Plastic Hearts* (2020), and *Endless Summer Vacation* (2023). Her single "Flowers" reached No. 1 on the Billboard Hot 100, became one of the most-streamed songs of 2023, and won Grammy Awards for Record of the Year and Best Pop Solo Performance. Across her career she has earned multiple No. 1 albums, Billboard Hot 100 hits, and major music awards while continuing acting and live touring.

Millie Mackintosh is a television personality, author, and entrepreneur who gained national recognition after appearing as a main cast member on the E4 reality series *Made in Chelsea* (2011–2013). She expanded into fashion and beauty by launching clothing collaborations and partnering with brands including Boots on licensed beauty products. In 2015 she published the lifestyle book *Made: A Book of Style, Food and Fitness*, extending her work into publishing. She later built a large social-media audience and developed business ventures and media projects in fashion, wellness, and lifestyle content. She has also co-authored *Bad Drunk: How I Found My Freedom from Alcohol and You Can Too* (2023) and continues to work across publishing, digital media, and brand partnerships.

Mohamed Salah is a professional soccer player who rose to prominence after joining Liverpool FC in 2017 and scoring 44 goals in his first season, including a then-record 32 in a 38-game Premier League campaign. After earlier spells with Basel, Chelsea, Fiorentina, and Roma, he established himself as Liverpool's leading scorer of the modern era, surpassing 200 goals for the club and becoming its all-time top scorer in Premier League competition. He has won the UEFA Champions League (2019), Premier League (2020), FA Cup, League Cups, and FIFA Club World Cup with Liverpool. Individually, he has earned multiple Premier League Golden Boots and African Footballer of the Year awards while maintaining consistent 20-plus-goal seasons across domestic and European competitions.

MrBeast (Jimmy Donaldson) is a digital creator and entrepreneur who first gained attention in 2017 after viral stunt videos on YouTube, including a video counting to 100,000. He launched his main YouTube channel in 2012 and expanded into large-scale challenge, philanthropy, and competition videos, becoming one of the platform's most-subscribed creators with hundreds of millions of subscribers across channels. He founded Beast Industries, which includes ventures such as MrBeast Burger (2020) and the snack brand Feastables (2022), distributed through major retail chains. His media company produces YouTube content, brand partnerships, and consumer products, generating substantial annual revenue and expanding into global distribution and entertainment ventures by the mid-2020s.

Muhammad Ali is a professional boxer and activist who became widely known after winning the Olympic light heavyweight gold medal in 1960 and defeating Sonny Liston to claim the world heavyweight title in 1964. Born Cassius Clay, he changed his name in 1964 after joining the Nation of Islam. In 1967 he refused induction into the U.S. Army, resulting in the loss of his titles and boxing license until the U.S. Supreme Court overturned his conviction in 1971. He regained the heavyweight championship by defeating George Foreman in 1974 and later became the first three-time lineal heavyweight champion after defeating Leon Spinks in 1978. His bouts against Joe Frazier and Foreman were global events, and he remained a public figure through humanitarian work until his death in 2016.

Naomi Campbell is a model and entrepreneur who rose to prominence in the late 1980s after appearing in major runway shows and fashion editorials worldwide. Discovered at 15 in London, she became the first Black model on the cover of *French Vogue* (1988) and later appeared on the September cover of *American Vogue* (1989) and the cover of *Time* (1991). She worked extensively with fashion houses including Chanel, Versace, Prada, and Louis Vuitton and appeared on hundreds of magazine covers. In 2005 she founded Fashion for Relief, a charity initiative that has raised funds for disaster relief and humanitarian causes through fashion events. She has also expanded into business ventures, television appearances, and fashion mentorship while remaining active in the industry for more than four decades.

Natalie Portman is an actor and filmmaker who first gained attention with her film debut in *Léon: The Professional* (1994) at age 12. She became widely known as Padmé Amidala in the *Star Wars* prequel trilogy (1999–2005), including *Revenge of the Sith*, which grossed over $800 million worldwide. She earned a Golden Globe and Academy Award nomination for *Closer* (2004) and later won the Academy Award for Best Actress for *Black Swan* (2010). She continued leading films such as *Jackie* (2016), which earned another Oscar nomination, and joined the Marvel Cinematic Universe as Jane Foster in the *Thor* series.

She has also directed and produced films, including *A Tale of Love and Darkness* (2015), expanding her work beyond acting.

Naval Ravikant is an entrepreneur and investor who co-founded Epinions in 1999, which later merged into Shopping.com and went public in 2004. He founded Venture Hacks in 2007 and co-founded AngelList in 2010, a platform connecting startups with investors, which later expanded into venture funds, talent recruiting, and startup infrastructure under AngelList Talent and AngelList Venture. As an angel investor, he backed early-stage companies including Twitter, Uber, Yammer, Stack Overflow, and Postmates. He co-founded MetaStable Capital in 2014, an early cryptocurrency hedge fund. In 2017 he launched Spearhead, a venture program backing founders as angel investors. His ideas gained wider readership through *The Almanack of Naval Ravikant* (2020), a curated collection of his writings and interviews.

Nick Saban is a football coach who became a college head coach at Toledo in 1990 before leading Michigan State and winning a BCS national championship at LSU in the 2003 season. He briefly coached the NFL's Miami Dolphins from 2005 to 2006, then took over Alabama in 2007 and won six national championships there, giving him seven total as a college head coach. His Alabama teams won nine SEC championships and made eight College Football Playoff appearances. He retired from coaching after the 2023 season with a career college head coaching record of 292–71–1. His programs produced multiple Heisman Trophy winners and numerous first-round NFL draft picks, and he later joined ESPN as a college football analyst.

Nicki Minaj is a rapper, singer, and songwriter who rose to prominence after releasing mixtapes between 2007 and 2009 before her debut album *Pink Friday* (2010) entered the Billboard 200 at No. 2 and was later certified multi-platinum. She followed with albums including *Pink Friday: Roman Reloaded* (2012), *The Pinkprint* (2014), *Queen* (2018), and *Pink Friday 2* (2023), earning multiple platinum certifications. Since 2010 she has accumulated more than 140 Billboard Hot 100 entries, including over 20 top-ten hits such as "Super Bass," "Starships," "Anaconda," and "Bang Bang." Her cumulative output includes over 100 million RIAA-certified units, placing her among the best-certified female rappers, and she has maintained chart presence across more than a decade of releases and collaborations.

Nikki Glaser is a stand-up comedian, actor, and television host who gained national recognition after appearing on NBC's *Last Comic Standing* in 2006 and 2007. She co-created and hosted MTV's *Nikki & Sara Live* (2013) and later hosted Comedy Central's *Not Safe with Nikki Glaser* (2016). Her stand-up specials include *Perfect* (2016), *Bangin'* (2019), *Good Clean Filth* (2022), and *Someday You'll Die* (2024). From 2018 to 2020 she hosted the SiriusXM morning show *You Up with Nikki Glaser* and later hosted HBO Max reality series *FBoy Island* (2021–2023). In 2025 she hosted the 82nd Golden Globe Awards, expanding her presence into major live awards broadcasting while maintaining touring, podcasting, and television projects.

Nikki Sixx is a bassist, songwriter, and radio host who co-founded Mötley Crüe in 1981 and served as its primary songwriter on albums including *Too Fast for Love, Shout at the Devil, Theatre of Pain, Girls, Girls, Girls*, and *Dr. Feelgood*. He wrote or co-wrote songs such as "Live Wire," "Home Sweet Home," "Kickstart My Heart," and "Dr. Feelgood," contributing to more than 100 million records sold worldwide by the band. He later formed Sixx:A.M., releasing multiple albums beginning in 2007, and co-authored *The Dirt* (2001), a bestselling band memoir later adapted into a 2019 Netflix film. Beyond performing, he hosted the syndicated radio show *Sixx Sense* (2010–2017) and participated in Mötley Crüe reunion tours and stadium performances into the 2020s.

Oksana Baiul is a figure skater who won the 1993 World Figure Skating Championships at age 15 and the 1994 Olympic gold medal in ladies' singles, becoming the first Olympic champion for independent Ukraine. She turned professional after the Olympics, moved to the United States, and toured for years with shows such as *Champions on Ice*, appearing in televised skating specials and exhibitions. In 1997 she published *Oksana: My Own Story* and *Secrets of Skating*. She later continued performing internationally and launched the Oksana Baiul Collection, a skating apparel line. In 2015 she settled a lawsuit with the

Ukrainian government regarding use of her name in skating venues. She has remained involved in skating exhibitions, brand licensing, and public appearances.

Patrick Swayze is an actor and dancer who rose to prominence in the 1980s through film, television, and stage roles. After early dance training and Broadway work, he gained recognition as Darrel Curtis in *The Outsiders* (1983) and in the miniseries *North and South* (1985–1986). He became a leading film star with *Dirty Dancing* (1987), whose soundtrack and global box office expanded his visibility, followed by *Ghost* (1990), one of the decade's highest-grossing films, earning him a Golden Globe nomination. He also starred in *Road House* (1989), *Point Break* (1991), and later appeared in *Donnie Darko* (2001). Diagnosed with pancreatic cancer in 2008, he completed the television series *The Beast* (2009) before his death on September 14, 2009.

Pharrell Williams is a musician, producer, and fashion designer who gained notoriety in the late 1990s as one half of The Neptunes production duo. With Chad Hugo, he produced major hits for artists including Jay-Z, Britney Spears, and Nelly, and co-founded the band N.E.R.D. He released solo albums *In My Mind* (2006) and *G I R L* (2014), whose single "Happy" became a global No. 1 hit, earned an Academy Award nomination, and became one of the best-selling songs of its era. He has won 13 Grammy Awards and contributed to multiple Billboard Hot 100 No. 1 singles as producer and performer. Beyond music, he co-founded Billionaire Boys Club and Ice Cream apparel brands and, in 2023, was appointed men's creative director at Louis Vuitton, expanding his influence into luxury fashion.

Pink (Alecia Moore) is a singer and songwriter who rose to celebrity with her 2000 debut album *Can't Take Me Home*, which was certified double platinum in the United States and produced Top 10 singles including "There You Go." She reached global No. 1 in 2001 with "Lady Marmalade," earning a Grammy Award, and expanded her audience with *Missundaztood* (2001), which sold over 13 million copies worldwide and produced hits such as "Get the Party Started." She has released multiple chart-topping albums including *I'm Not Dead*, *Funhouse*, *The Truth About Love*, *Beautiful Trauma*, and *Trustfall*.

Across her career she has sold over 90 million records worldwide, won three Grammy Awards, and sustained major global touring success with several of the highest-grossing arena tours of their years.

Raymond Carver is a short-story writer and poet who gained national distinction with his debut collection *Will You Please Be Quiet, Please?* (1976), a National Book Award finalist that established his reputation in contemporary fiction. He followed with *What We Talk About When We Talk About Love* (1981), which became associated with minimalist American prose, and expanded his narrative range in *Cathedral* (1983), a Pulitzer Prize finalist. His final major collection, *Where I'm Calling From* (1988), compiled earlier and new stories shortly before his death. In addition to fiction, he published several poetry collections and taught at universities including Syracuse. His stories appeared in major literary magazines such as *Esquire* and *The New Yorker*, and his work influenced late-20th-century short fiction.

Rebecca West is a novelist, journalist, critic, and travel writer who gained recognition in the 1910s through suffrage journalism and literary criticism, including early essays on Henry James. She published her debut novel *The Return of the Soldier* in 1918, establishing her literary reputation. She later produced novels, biography, and political reportage while contributing criticism to major British and American publications. Her travel study *Black Lamb and Grey Falcon* (1941), based on prewar journeys in Yugoslavia, became a major English-language work on Balkan history and culture. After World War II she reported on the Nuremberg trials in *The Meaning of Treason* (1947) and *A Train of Powder* (1955). She continued publishing fiction and criticism into the 1960s, and her writings have remained in print and scholarly circulation.

Rich Roll is an ultra-endurance athlete, author, and podcast host who transitioned from collegiate swimming and entertainment law into endurance competition and media. After swimming at Stanford and earning a law degree from Cornell, he worked in entertainment law before turning to ultra-endurance sports in his late 30s. He completed the Ultraman World Championships and, in 2010, finished the EPIC5 Challenge: five Ironman-distance triathlons on five Hawaiian islands in five days. His memoir *Finding Ultra* (2012) became a bestseller and expanded his public profile. He launched *The Rich Roll Podcast* in 2012, which grew into a long-running interview show featuring athletes, scientists, and public figures, reaching a global audience through podcast platforms and digital media.

Rick Rubin is a record producer and label founder who co-founded Def Jam Recordings in 1984 while a student at NYU, producing early releases for artists including LL Cool J, Run-D.M.C., and Beastie Boys. He founded American Recordings in 1988, working with artists such as Slayer and producing Johnny Cash's *American Recordings* series beginning in 1994. He produced Red Hot Chili Peppers' *Blood Sugar Sex Magik* (1991) and *Californication* (1999), and later projects with Metallica, Jay-Z, Adele, and others. He has won multiple Grammy Awards, including Producer of the Year and Album of the Year credits. In 2023 he published *The Creative Act: A Way of Being*, a bestselling book on creativity drawn from his production philosophy and decades of studio work.

Ringo Starr is a musician, singer, songwriter, and actor who joined the Beatles in August 1962, replacing Pete Best and performing on all their subsequent recordings and tours. He sang lead vocals on songs including "With a Little Help from My Friends," "Yellow Submarine," and "Octopus's Garden," and contributed as a songwriter. After the Beatles disbanded in 1970, he released solo hits such as "Photograph," "It Don't Come Easy," and "You're Sixteen," with his 1973 album *Ringo* reaching No. 2 in the U.S. He launched the All-Starr Band in 1989, touring internationally with rotating lineups. He has won multiple Grammy Awards, was inducted into the Rock and Roll Hall of Fame with the Beatles and as a solo artist, and was knighted in 2018.

Rob Lowe is an actor, producer, and podcast host who rose to prominence in films such as *The Outsiders* (1983), *St. Elmo's Fire* (1985), and *About Last Night...* (1986), becoming associated with the "Brat Pack." He later earned Emmy and Golden Globe nominations for his role as Sam Seaborn on *The West Wing* (1999–2003). He went on to star in television series including *Brothers & Sisters*, *Parks and Recreation*, and *9-1-1: Lone Star* (2020–2023). He authored the memoirs *Stories I Only Tell My Friends* (2011) and *Love Life* (2014), both New York Times bestsellers. Since 2020 he has hosted the podcast *Literally! with Rob Lowe* and continued acting in film and television, sustaining a screen and media career spanning more than four decades.

Robbie Williams is a singer-songwriter who gained national fame as a member of Take That from 1990 to 1995, contributing to multiple UK number-one singles and albums. After leaving the group, he launched a solo career with *Life Thru a Lens* (1997), whose single "Angels" became a signature hit. He followed with chart-topping albums including *I've Been Expecting You* (1998), *Sing When You're Winning* (2000), *Swing When You're Winning* (2001), and *Escapology* (2002). His solo releases have sold over 75 million records worldwide, and he has achieved 14 UK number-one albums, among the most for a solo artist. He has won 18 BRIT Awards and continued touring globally, releasing new music and appearing in the Netflix docuseries *Robbie Williams* (2023).

Robin Williams is an actor and comedian who achieved early celebrity as the alien Mork on the television series *Mork & Mindy* (1978–1982). He transitioned to film with acclaimed performances in *Good Morning, Vietnam* (1987), *Dead Poets Society* (1989), and *The Fisher King* (1991), earning Academy Award nominations for each. During the 1990s he appeared in major films including *Aladdin* (1992), voicing the Genie, *Mrs. Doubtfire* (1993), *Jumanji* (1995), and *Good Will Hunting* (1997), winning the Academy Award for Best Supporting Actor for the latter. He also maintained a stand-up career and television appearances. Across film, television, and comedy, he received an Academy Award, two Emmy Awards, six Golden Globe Awards, and five Grammy Awards.

Ronda Rousey is a mixed martial artist, professional wrestler, and judoka who became the first American woman to win an Olympic judo medal, earning bronze at the 2008 Beijing Games. She transitioned to mixed martial arts in 2010, won the Strikeforce women's bantamweight title, and joined the UFC in 2012 as its first female fighter and inaugural women's bantamweight champion, defending the title six times. She compiled a 12–2 professional MMA record and was inducted into the UFC Hall of Fame in 2018. That year she debuted in WWE at WrestleMania 34, later winning the Raw Women's Championship and headlining WrestleMania 35 in the first women's main event. She also held the WWE SmackDown Women's Championship before stepping away from full-time wrestling.

Ruby Warrington is an author and journalist who established her career in London fashion and lifestyle media, including serving as features editor at *The Sunday Times Style*. In 2012 she founded the online magazine *The Numinous*, focused on contemporary spirituality and wellness culture. She published *Sober Curious* (2018), introducing a widely adopted term and concept, followed by *The Sober Curious Reset* (2020). She later authored *Material Girl, Mystical World* (2022) and *Women Without Kids* (2023), expanding into cultural commentary and lifestyle topics. In addition to writing, she works as a publishing consultant and "book doula," advising authors on manuscript development, positioning, and publishing strategy, extending her influence across contemporary nonfiction and publishing advisory work.

Rumer Willis is an actor and singer who began appearing in films as a child, including *Now and Then* (1995), *Striptease* (1996), and *Hostage* (2005). She later appeared in films such as *The House Bunny* (2008) and *Sorority Row* (2009) and had a recurring role on the CW series *90210* (2009–2010). In 2015 she won season 20 of *Dancing with the Stars* and made her Broadway debut as Roxie Hart in *Chicago*. She expanded into television with recurring roles on *Empire* and appearances in *Once Upon a Time in Hollywood* (2019). Alongside acting, she has performed as a singer in cabaret productions and live shows, developing a parallel career in music and stage performance.

RuPaul is a drag performer, television host, producer, singer, writer, and actor who gained international visibility with the 1993 album *Supermodel of the World* and its single "Supermodel (You Better Work)," which reached the Billboard Hot 100. He became a MAC Cosmetics spokesmodel and appeared in films and television during the 1990s. In 2009 he created, executive produced, and began hosting

RuPaul's Drag Race, which has run for more than 15 U.S. seasons and generated numerous international versions. He has won multiple Primetime Emmy Awards for Outstanding Host for a Reality or Competition Program and executive producing. He later launched talk shows, published books, and expanded World of Wonder productions. In 2018 he received a star on the Hollywood Walk of Fame, the first drag performer honored.

Russell Brand is a comedian, actor, author, and broadcaster who gained attention in the early 2000s through UK stand-up and television presenting, including hosting on MTV UK. He became internationally known for portraying Aldous Snow in *Forgetting Sarah Marshall* (2008) and *Get Him to the Greek* (2010), and for voicing Dr. Nefario in the *Despicable Me* film series. He hosted radio and television programs including *The Russell Brand Show* on BBC Radio 2 and Channel 4 projects. He is the author of several books, including memoirs and works on politics and culture. In 2017, he launched the interview podcast *Under the Skin*, expanding his work into long-form digital broadcasting and online media.

Ryan Holiday is an author, media strategist, and founder of Brass Check who left college at 19 to apprentice with Robert Greene and later became director of marketing at American Apparel. Through his agency, he has advised companies, organizations, and authors on media strategy. His first book, *Trust Me, I'm Lying* (2012), examined online media manipulation and became a Wall Street Journal bestseller. He later wrote books on Stoicism including *The Obstacle Is the Way* (2014), *Ego Is the Enemy* (2016), *The Daily Stoic* (2016), *Stillness Is the Key* (2019), and the Stoic Virtues series beginning with *Courage Is Calling* (2021). His books have sold millions of copies and been translated into dozens of languages.

Sadio Mané is a professional soccer player who became widely known after moving from Metz to Red Bull Salzburg, then joining Southampton in 2014. In May 2015 he set the Premier League record for the fastest hat-trick, scoring three times in 2 minutes 56 seconds against Aston Villa. He played for Liverpool from 2016 to 2022, scoring 120 goals in 269 appearances and winning the UEFA Champions

League (2019) and the Premier League (2019–20). He joined Bayern Munich in 2022, then moved to Al Nassr in 2023. For Senegal, he has been the national team's record goal scorer, won the Africa Cup of Nations in 2022, and was named CAF African Player of the Year in 2019 and 2022.

Samuel L. Jackson is an actor and producer who first gained attention with roles including Mister Señor Love Daddy in *Do the Right Thing* (1989), Stacks Edwards in *Goodfellas* (1990), and Ray Arnold in *Jurassic Park* (1993). He became widely known after playing Jules Winnfield in *Pulp Fiction* (1994), earning an Academy Award nomination for Best Supporting Actor. His later films include *Die Hard with a Vengeance* (1995), *A Time to Kill* (1996), *Unbreakable* (2000), and *Shaft* (2000). He portrayed Mace Windu in the *Star Wars* prequel trilogy (1999–2005) and has played Nick Fury in Marvel projects since first appearing as the character in 2008.

Sanaa Lathan is an actor and director who first drew wide attention for *Love & Basketball* (2000), winning an NAACP Image Award for Outstanding Actress in a Motion Picture. Her film roles include *The Best Man* (1999), *Brown Sugar* (2002), *Alien vs. Predator* (2004), *Something New* (2006), and *Now You See Me 2* (2016). She received a 2004 Tony Award nomination for Best Featured Actress in a Play for *A Raisin in the Sun*. She voiced Donna Tubbs on *The Cleveland Show* (2009–2013) and *Family Guy*. She starred in Netflix's *Nappily Ever After* (2018) and earned a Primetime Emmy nomination for Outstanding Guest Actress in a Drama Series for *Succession* (2022). She made her feature directing debut with *On the Come Up* (2022).

Sarah Hepola is an author, journalist, and podcast host who became widely known after publishing the memoir *Blackout: Remembering the Things I Drank to Forget* (2015), a New York Times bestseller. She has worked as a writer and editor, including roles at the *Austin Chronicle*, *Dallas Observer*, and *Salon*, and her essays have appeared in outlets including *The New York Times Magazine*, *The Atlantic*, *Elle*, *Bloomberg Businessweek*, *The Guardian*, and *Texas Monthly*. She created and hosted Texas Monthly's narrative podcast *America's Girls*, an eight-part series on the Dallas Cowboys Cheerleaders. She co-hosts the weekly culture podcast *Smoke 'Em If You Got 'Em* with Nancy Rommelmann, and she has been a staff writer at *The Dallas Morning News*.

Sarah Jane Clarke is a fashion designer, entrepreneur, and wellness coach who first entered the public spotlight in 1999 after co-founding the label sass & bide with Heidi Middleton, beginning with a Portobello Road market stall and a reported A$70,000 start-up loan. The brand expanded internationally and presented collections at Australian Fashion Week as well as London and New York Fashion Weeks in the early 2000s. Myer took a controlling stake in sass & bide in 2011 and completed its acquisition in 2013; Clarke and Middleton exited the business in 2014. After a multi-year sabbatical, Clarke launched her eponymous label, SARAH-JANE CLARKE, in 2018, focused on travel-oriented capsule collections and digital brand content.

Shania Twain is a singer-songwriter who rose to prominence in the mid-1990s after her second album, *The Woman in Me* (1995), became a major commercial breakthrough and won the Grammy for Best Country Album. *Come On Over* (1997) became the best-selling country album and the best-selling studio album by a solo female artist, with worldwide sales reported at over 40 million and 12 singles including "You're Still the One" and "Man! I Feel Like a Woman!" With *Up!* (2002), she became the only woman with three consecutive RIAA Diamond-certified albums. After returning with *Now* (2017), she released *Queen of Me* (2023) and continued touring, including a Las Vegas residency, *Come On Over – All The Hits* (2024–2025).

Shawn Ryan is a podcast host and former U.S. Navy SEAL who served with SEAL Team 2 and SEAL Team 8 and later worked as a security contractor with Blackwater's Global Response Staff supporting CIA protective operations. He founded Vigilance Elite, a tactical training and media company, and in 2019 launched *The Shawn Ryan Show*, an interview program distributed on YouTube and major audio platforms. The show features military veterans, intelligence and national-security figures, journalists, and public officials, and it has been listed among Spotify's most-listened-to podcasts in the United States. Guests have included Donald Trump and Erik Prince.

Shia LaBeouf is an actor, writer, and director who first gained attention as Louis Stevens on Disney Channel's *Even Stevens* (2000–2003), winning a Daytime Emmy Award in 2003. His early film leads included *Holes* (2003) and *Disturbia* (2007), followed by franchise roles as Sam Witwicky in *Transformers* (2007), *Transformers: Revenge of the Fallen* (2009), and *Transformers: Dark of the Moon* (2011), and as Mutt Williams in *Indiana Jones and the Kingdom of the Crystal Skull* (2008). He later focused on independent films including *American Honey* (2016), *The Peanut Butter Falcon* (2019), and *Honey Boy* (2019), which he wrote. In 2022 he starred in Abel Ferrara's *Padre Pio* and was confirmed in the Catholic Church in 2023.

Sia is a singer-songwriter and producer who first entered the public spotlight with solo albums in the late 1990s and early 2000s and as a vocalist for the group Zero 7. She later achieved global success writing and featuring on songs including "Titanium" with David Guetta, "Wild Ones" with Flo Rida, and "Diamonds," recorded by Rihanna. Her album *1000 Forms of Fear* (2014), featuring the single "Chandelier," debuted at No. 1 on the Billboard 200 and earned Grammy nominations. She followed with *This Is Acting* (2016) and the hit singles "Cheap Thrills" and "Unstoppable." She has received multiple ARIA and APRA Music Awards, MTV Video Music Awards, and numerous Grammy Award nominations.

Slash (Saul Hudson) is a guitarist, songwriter, and bandleader who joined Guns N' Roses in 1985 and recorded *Appetite for Destruction* (1987) and *Use Your Illusion I* and *II* (1991), which included songs such as "Sweet Child o' Mine," "Welcome to the Jungle," and "November Rain." After leaving Guns N' Roses in 1996, he led Slash's Snakepit and co-founded Velvet Revolver; their debut album *Contraband* (2004) debuted at No. 1 on the Billboard 200, and the band won a Grammy for "Slither." From 2010 he released solo albums and records with Myles Kennedy and the Conspirators. He rejoined Guns N' Roses in 2016 for the *Not in This Lifetime... Tour* and was inducted into the Rock and Roll Hall of Fame with the band in 2012.

Soko (Stéphanie Sokolinski) is a singer-songwriter and actor who gained international recognition with her 2007 debut single "I'll Kill Her," which became a major radio hit across Europe and topped Denmark's music charts. She released the albums *I Thought I Was an Alien* (2012), produced by Ross Robinson, *My Dreams Dictate My Reality* (2015), and *Feel Feelings* (2020), establishing an international indie music career. As an actor, she has appeared in acclaimed films including *In the Beginning* (2009), *Augustine* (2012), and *The Dancer* (2016), which premiered at the Cannes Film Festival, where she portrayed dancer Loïe Fuller. Her work spans music, film, and international touring.

Stephen King is a novelist and short-story writer who first gained attention after his debut novel *Carrie* (1974) became a bestseller and was adapted into a successful film. He followed with *'Salem's Lot* (1975) and *The Shining* (1977), and later wrote major works including *The Stand*, *It*, *Misery*, *The Green Mile*, and the eight-volume *Dark Tower* series. He also authored the memoir *On Writing* (2000), *11/22/63* (2011), the Bill Hodges trilogy (2014–2016), and later novels including *Fairy Tale* (2022) and *Holly* (2023). His books have sold more than 350 million copies worldwide. He received the National Book Foundation Medal for Distinguished Contribution to American Letters (2003) and the National Medal of Arts (2015).

Steve Harvey is a comedian, actor, author, radio personality, and television host who achieved celebrity after becoming host of *It's Showtime at the Apollo* (1993–2000). He starred in *The Steve Harvey Show* (1996–2002) and was featured in *The Original Kings of Comedy* tour and Spike Lee's 2000 concert film. He launched *The Steve Harvey Morning Show* in 2000, which became nationally syndicated. In 2010 he became host of *Family Feud*, later becoming its longest-serving host. He also hosted the daytime talk show *Steve Harvey* (2012–2017) and later *Judge Steve Harvey* (2022–2024). He has received multiple Daytime Emmy Awards and NAACP Image Awards and was honored with a star on the Hollywood Walk of Fame in 2013.

Steve-O (Stephen Glover) is a stunt performer, comedian, author, and podcast host who became widely known as a core cast member of

MTV's *Jackass* (2000–2002) and its subsequent film series. He co-starred in the spin-off series *Wildboyz* (2003–2006) and later performed in live comedy and stunt tours. He published the memoir *Professional Idiot* (2011), which became a New York Times bestseller. He has released stand-up comedy specials and continues touring internationally. In 2020 he launched the interview podcast *Wild Ride! with Steve-O*, distributed on YouTube and audio platforms, expanding his work into digital media and long-form interviews.

Steve Sarkisian is a football coach and former quarterback who began his coaching career at USC in the early 2000s, contributing to multiple conference championships and a national title during the program's peak years. He became head coach at Washington (2009–2013) and later USC (2014–2015). He then served as offensive coordinator at Alabama, helping lead the team to a 13–0 season and College Football Playoff national championship in 2020, and received the Broyles Award as the nation's top assistant coach. He was hired as head coach at Texas in 2021 and led the program to consecutive 12-win seasons in 2023 and 2024, including a conference championship and College Football Playoff appearances.

Steven Bartlett is an entrepreneur, investor, author, and podcast host who entered the public spotlight in the mid-2010s after co-founding the social-media marketing company Social Chain in 2014. In 2019, Social Chain combined with a Germany-listed company and traded publicly as The Social Chain AG. He launched *The Diary of a CEO* podcast in 2017; in 2024 it was reported to have surpassed 1 billion streams across major platforms, and Spotify Wrapped listed it among the world's most-listened-to podcasts in 2025. In 2021 he joined BBC's *Dragons' Den* as an investor. He later founded Flight Story and Flight Fund and co-founded the web3 developer platform thirdweb, and he is associated with the venture Steven.com.

Steven Tyler is a singer and songwriter who became widely known as the frontman of Aerosmith, leading the band's breakthrough era with albums including *Toys in the Attic* (1975) and *Rocks* (1976) and songs such as "Dream On," "Sweet Emotion," and "Walk This Way." He fronted Aerosmith's late-1980s and 1990s commercial resurgence with multi-platinum albums including *Permanent Vacation* (1987), *Pump* (1989), *Get a Grip* (1993), and *Nine Lives* (1997). Aerosmith has sold more than 150 million records worldwide and was inducted into the Rock & Roll Hall of Fame in 2001. Tyler served as a judge on *American Idol* (2011–2012) and released the solo album *We're All Somebody from Somewhere* (2016). Aerosmith announced retirement from touring in 2024.

Sugar Ray Leonard is a boxer and Olympic gold medalist who won National Golden Gloves titles in 1973 and 1974, AAU national championships in 1974 and 1975, and gold at the 1975 Pan American Games before winning the 1976 Olympic light-welterweight title. Turning professional in 1977, he won world championships in five weight divisions—welterweight, light middleweight, middleweight, super middleweight, and light heavyweight—and earned signature victories over Wilfred Benítez, Roberto Durán, Thomas Hearns, and Marvin Hagler. He retired with a 36–3–1 record (25 knockouts) and was inducted into the International Boxing Hall of Fame in 1997.

Terry Crews is an actor, television host, and former NFL player who was drafted by the Los Angeles Rams in 1991 and later played for the Rams, San Diego Chargers, and Washington Redskins, along with a 1995 season in NFL Europe with Rhein Fire; he left professional football in 1997. He transitioned into entertainment as "T-Money" on *Battle Dome* (1999–2001) and later appeared in films including *The 6th Day* (2000), *White Chicks* (2004), *The Longest Yard* (2005), and *The Expendables* series (2010–2014). On television he starred in *Everybody Hates Chris* (2005–2009) and *Brooklyn Nine-Nine* (2013–2021) and became a long-running face of Old Spice campaigns. Since 2019 he has hosted *America's Got Talent*.

Theo Fleury is a hockey right wing and Stanley Cup champion who debuted with the Calgary Flames in 1988–89, recording 34 points in 36 regular-season games and helping win the 1989 Stanley Cup. Across 1,084 NHL games with Calgary, Colorado, the New York Rangers, and Chicago, he totaled 455 goals and 633 assists (1,088 points), plus 79 points in 77 playoff games. Internationally, he won gold with Canada at the 1996 World Cup of Hockey and earned Olympic gold at the 2002

Winter Olympics after also appearing at the 1998 Games. He later played professionally in Europe, including a stint with the Belfast Giants, before retiring.

Theo Von is a stand-up comedian, podcaster, and former reality TV personality who first gained visibility on MTV's *Road Rules: Maximum Velocity Tour* (2000) and multiple seasons of *The Challenge* in the early 2000s. After moving to Los Angeles, he won the viewer-voted online competition *Last Comic Downloaded* tied to *Last Comic Standing* (2006). He released the Netflix stand-up special *Theo Von: No Offense* (2016) and the comedy album *30lb Bag of Hamster Bones* (2017), followed by the Netflix special *Theo Von: Regular People* (2021). He hosted Yahoo's *Primetime in No Time* and the TBS hidden-camera series *Deal With It* (2013–2014). He hosts the long-running podcast *This Past Weekend* and co-hosted *The King and the Sting* (2018–2022).

Theodore Roosevelt is a statesman and political leader who became the 26th president of the United States (1901–1909) after serving briefly as vice president under William McKinley. He gained national prominence leading the Rough Riders during the Spanish–American War and was elected governor of New York in 1898. As president, he pursued antitrust enforcement, supported federal regulation of railroads and food and drug safety, mediated the 1902 coal strike, and expanded national forests, parks, and monuments. He supported construction of the Panama Canal and expansion of the U.S. Navy. In 1912 he ran for president as the Progressive Party nominee, winning 88 electoral votes and finishing second in the election.

Tim Allen is a stand-up comedian and actor who became widely known starring in the ABC sitcom *Home Improvement* (1991–1999), winning a Golden Globe Award and multiple People's Choice Awards. In 1994 he starred in the film *The Santa Clause*, which became a box office success, and published the bestselling book *Don't Stand Too Close to a Naked Man*. He voiced Buzz Lightyear in the *Toy Story* film series beginning in 1995. He later starred in the sitcom *Last Man Standing* (2011–2021) and reprised his role in *The Santa Clauses* television series (2022–2023). He received a star on the Hollywood Walk of Fame in 2004 and was named a Disney Legend in 2009.

Tim McGraw is a country recording artist and actor who rose to prominence with his breakthrough album *Not a Moment Too Soon* (1994), the best-selling country album of that year. He has released 17 studio albums, including multiple No. 1 titles on the Billboard Top Country Albums chart. His singles include 25 Billboard Hot Country Songs No. 1 hits such as "It's Your Love," "Just to See You Smile," and "Live Like You Were Dying." He has sold tens of millions of records worldwide and received three Grammy Awards along with numerous ACM and CMA Awards. He has continued releasing albums, including *Standing Room Only* (2023), and touring internationally into the 2020s.

Tim Tebow is a quarterback and broadcaster who gained national fame at the University of Florida, becoming the first sophomore to win the Heisman Trophy (2007) and helping the team win BCS national championships in 2006 and 2008. He was selected in the first round of the 2010 NFL Draft by the Denver Broncos and led the team to a division title and playoff victory during the 2011 season. He later played for the New York Jets and pursued additional NFL opportunities. From 2016 to 2021 he played in Minor League Baseball in the New York Mets organization. He joined ESPN's SEC Network as a college football analyst and founded the Tim Tebow Foundation, which operates international charitable programs including Night to Shine.

Tom Bilyeu is an entrepreneur and media host who co-founded Quest Nutrition in 2010, helping build it into a widely distributed protein-bar company. Quest Nutrition was acquired by The Simply Good Foods Company in 2019 in a transaction valued at approximately $1 billion. After stepping away from Quest, he founded Impact Theory, a media and content studio focused on interviews and educational programming. Through Impact Theory, he hosts long-form interview series and develops content for entrepreneurs and business audiences across YouTube and digital platforms. He has also launched courses and business education programs through the Impact Theory platform.

Tom Cruise is an actor and producer who became widely known after breakout roles in *Risky Business* (1983) and *Top Gun* (1986). He starred in films including *Rain Man* (1988), *A Few Good Men* (1992), and *Jerry Maguire* (1996), earning three Academy Award nominations for acting. In 1996 he launched and produced the *Mission: Impossible* film series, returning through *Dead Reckoning Part One* (2023) and *The Final Reckoning* (2025). He reprised his role in *Top Gun: Maverick* (2022), which grossed more than $1.45 billion worldwide and earned a Best Picture nomination as a production. He received an Honorary Academy Award in 2025.

Tom Felton is an actor who became widely known after being cast as Draco Malfoy in all eight *Harry Potter* films (2001–2011). He appeared earlier in *The Borrowers* (1997) and *Anna and the King* (1999). For his work as Draco Malfoy, he won MTV Movie Awards for Best Villain in 2010 and 2011. After the film series, he acted in projects including *Rise of the Planet of the Apes* (2011) and *The Flash* (2016–2017). He published the memoir *Beyond the Wand: The Magic and Mayhem of Growing Up a Wizard* (2022). In 2025 he made his Broadway debut, reprising Draco Malfoy in *Harry Potter and the Cursed Child*.

Tom Ford is a fashion designer and filmmaker who became a leading luxury creative director at Gucci (1994–2004) and also led Yves Saint Laurent's ready-to-wear as creative director after Gucci acquired the house (1999–2004). In 2005 he launched the TOM FORD brand, expanding from beauty and eyewear into menswear, womenswear, accessories, and retail boutiques. In 2023, The Estée Lauder Companies completed the acquisition of the TOM FORD brand in a deal valued at about $2.8 billion, with Zegna acquiring the TOM FORD FASHION business. He wrote and directed the feature films *A Single Man* (2009) and *Nocturnal Animals* (2016).

Tom Holland is an actor who became widely known after debuting onstage in London's West End in *Billy Elliot the Musical* (2008) and moving into film with *The Impossible* (2012). He later appeared in *How I Live Now* (2013) and *In the Heart of the Sea* (2015). In 2016 he joined the Marvel Cinematic Universe as Peter Parker/Spider-Man in *Captain America: Civil War*, then led three *Spider-Man* films (2017–2021) and appeared in *Avengers* ensemble films (2018–2019). He headlined projects including *The Devil All the Time* (2020), *Cherry* (2021), *Uncharted* (2022), and Apple TV+'s *The Crowded Room* (2023). He won the BAFTA Rising Star Award (2017) and returned to the West End in 2024 as Romeo in *Romeo & Juliet*.

Tom Segura is a stand-up comedian, writer, and podcast host who first gained wider attention through TV appearances including *Live at Gotham* and *Comedy Central Presents*. He released stand-up specials including *Completely Normal* (2014), Netflix's *Mostly Stories* (2016), *Disgraceful* (2018), *Ball Hog* (2020), *Sledgehammer* (2023), and Netflix's *Teacher* (2025). In 2010 he co-created the comedy podcast *Your Mom's House* with Christina Pazsitzky and expanded it into YMH Studios, which has produced series including *2 Bears 1 Cave*, *Dr. Drew After Dark*, and *Where My Moms At*. He published the essay collection *I'd Like to Play Alone, Please* (2022) and continues touring internationally.

Tony Adams is a soccer defender who became widely known after debuting for Arsenal in 1983 and becoming the club's captain at age 21 in 1988. He spent his entire senior club career with Arsenal (1983–2002), making 669 appearances and captaining the team to four league titles (1988–89, 1990–91, 1997–98, 2001–02), three FA Cups, two League Cups, and the 1994 European Cup Winners' Cup. He also captained England and represented the national team at major tournaments. After retiring from professional football, he founded Sporting Chance, an organization that provides residential and outpatient support services for athletes and sports professionals.

Tony Dungy is an NFL head coach and former safety who became head coach of the Tampa Bay Buccaneers in 1996, leading the team to four playoff appearances and helping establish the Tampa 2 defensive system. He was hired by the Indianapolis Colts in 2002 and led the team to seven consecutive playoff appearances and victory in Super Bowl XLI, becoming the first Black head coach to win a Super Bowl. Across 13 seasons as a head coach, he compiled a 139–69 regular-season record and reached the postseason 11 times. After retiring from coaching in 2009, he joined NBC Sports as an NFL analyst and authored several books. He was inducted into the Pro Football Hall of Fame in 2016.

Tony Robbins is a speaker, author, and business owner who entered the public spotlight in the 1980s through seminars, infomercials, and personal-development programs. He created multi-day events including *Unleash the Power Within*, which expanded internationally and into digital formats. He authored bestselling books including *Awaken the Giant Within* (1991), *Money: Master the Game* (2014), and *Unshakeable* (2017). He founded and invested in companies across industries including financial services, hospitality, media, and coaching. Over several decades he has hosted seminars, produced educational content, and appeared in television, streaming, and live productions.

Travis Barker is a drummer and producer who became widely known after joining Blink-182 in 1998 and recording *Enema of the State* (1999), which brought the band mainstream success. He continued with Blink-182 on albums including *Take Off Your Pants and Jacket* (2001), *Blink-182* (2003), *California* (2016), and *One More Time…* (2023). He also formed and performed with Box Car Racer, +44, and Transplants. In addition to band work, he collaborated with artists across rock, hip-hop, and pop and released the solo album *Give the Drummer Some* (2011). He has continued touring internationally with Blink-182 and recording collaborative projects.

Trent Reznor is a songwriter, producer, and bandleader who founded Nine Inch Nails in 1988 and wrote and recorded the debut album *Pretty Hate Machine* (1989). He achieved mainstream success with *The Downward Spiral* (1994) and *The Fragile* (1999), both certified multi-platinum. He founded Nothing Records and later released Nine Inch Nails projects including *Ghosts I–IV* and *The Slip* (2008). In collaboration with Atticus Ross, he became a film composer and won the Academy Award for Best Original Score for *The Social Network* (2010), followed by additional Academy Awards and Golden Globe Awards. He was inducted into the Rock and Roll Hall of Fame as a member of Nine Inch Nails in 2020.

Trey Anastasio is a guitarist, composer, and bandleader who co-founded Phish in 1983 and developed the group's catalog as a primary songwriter and performer. He contributed to albums including *Junta* (1989), *Billy Breathes* (1996), and *Farmhouse* (2000), and led major live performances including Phish's 13-show "Baker's Dozen" residency at Madison Square Garden in 2017. He released multiple solo albums and formed projects including Trey Anastasio Band and Oysterhead. He also composed the score for the Broadway musical *Hands on a Hardbody* (2013), earning a Tony Award nomination. In addition to his music career, he founded the Divided Sky Foundation, which operates a residential recovery and support facility in Vermont.

Truett Cathy is a fast-food founder who opened the Dwarf Grill in Hapeville, Georgia, in 1946 and later developed the chicken sandwich that became the signature item of Chick-fil-A. In 1967 he opened the first Chick-fil-A restaurant in Atlanta's Greenbriar Shopping Center, pioneering mall-based fast-food locations. The company expanded to freestanding restaurants and grew to thousands of locations across the United States. He established the WinShape Foundation in 1984 to support scholarships, education, and youth programs. He led Chick-fil-A as a privately held, family-run company for decades until his death in 2014.

Tucker Carlson is a television host, author, and commentator who became a central primetime figure in American cable news as host of CNN's *Crossfire* (2001–2005) and later *Tucker Carlson Tonight* on Fox News (2016–2023). He co-founded the news and commentary company *The Daily Caller* in 2010 and served as editor-in-chief until 2020. His Fox News program became the highest-rated cable news broadcast in the United States for multiple consecutive years. After departing the network in 2023, he launched independent interview and commentary programming distributed directly through online platforms, reaching a large global audience and continuing his long-running media career.

Tyler Perry is a writer, actor, director, and producer who built an independent film and television enterprise based on characters he created, including Madea. Beginning with touring stage plays in the

1990s, he self-financed his first film, *Diary of a Mad Black Woman* (2005), which became a box office success. He went on to create more than 20 feature films and television series including *House of Payne*, *Meet the Browns*, and *The Oval*, while retaining ownership of his productions. In 2019 he opened Tyler Perry Studios in Atlanta, a 330-acre production facility used for film and television projects. He has also produced content through major distribution agreements across film, television, and streaming platforms.

Tyler the Creator is a rapper, producer, and designer who co-founded the Odd Future collective and released his debut mixtape *Bastard* (2009), followed by the studio album *Goblin* (2011), which included the single "Yonkers." He later released albums including *Wolf* (2013), *Cherry Bomb* (2015), *Flower Boy* (2017), *Igor* (2019), and *Call Me If You Get Lost* (2021). *Igor* and *Call Me If You Get Lost* each won the Grammy Award for Best Rap Album. He founded the Golf Wang clothing brand and created the Camp Flog Gnaw Carnival music festival. His work spans music, fashion, and media, with international tours and ongoing creative projects.

Tyra Banks is a model, producer, television host, and entrepreneur who became widely known in the 1990s as one of the original Victoria's Secret Angels and the first Black woman to appear solo on the covers of *GQ* and the *Sports Illustrated Swimsuit Issue*. In 2003 she created and hosted *America's Next Top Model*, which ran for 24 cycles and was distributed internationally. She also hosted *The Tyra Banks Show* (2005–2010), winning two Daytime Emmy Awards. She later hosted *America's Got Talent* (2017–2018) and *Dancing with the Stars* (2020–2022). She founded Bankable Productions, launched Tyra Beauty, and created the SMiZE & DREAM ice cream brand.

Tyson Fury is a heavyweight boxer who became world champion by defeating Wladimir Klitschko in 2015 to win the WBA, IBF, WBO, IBO, and lineal heavyweight titles. After returning to competition in 2018, he fought Deontay Wilder to a draw and then defeated him in 2020 to win the WBC heavyweight championship, successfully defending it in their 2021 trilogy bout. He unified major heavyweight titles during his career and headlined major events in the United Kingdom and United

States. He later fought Oleksandr Usyk in 2024 and 2025 in bouts for the undisputed heavyweight championship.

Ulysses S. Grant is a military officer and political leader who commanded Union armies to victory in the Civil War and later served as the 18th president of the United States (1869–1877). A West Point graduate, he captured Forts Henry and Donelson (1862), led the Union victory at Vicksburg (1863), and as General-in-Chief accepted Robert E. Lee's surrender at Appomattox (1865). As president, he enforced Reconstruction laws, including federal measures to protect voting rights and suppress Ku Klux Klan violence. After leaving office, he wrote *Personal Memoirs of Ulysses S. Grant* (1885), which became a widely read military autobiography.

Valerie Bertinelli is an actor, television host, and author who became widely known as Barbara Cooper on the sitcom *One Day at a Time* (1975–1984), winning two Golden Globe Awards. She later starred in the series *Hot in Cleveland* (2010–2015). She published memoirs including *Losing It: And Gaining My Life Back One Pound at a Time* (2008), which became a bestseller. She created and hosted *Valerie's Home Cooking* (2015–2023) and co-hosted *Kids Baking Championship* on Food Network, winning two Daytime Emmy Awards. She also published several cookbooks and lifestyle titles.

Virat Kohli is a cricket batter who became captain of India's Under-19 team and led them to the ICC Under-19 World Cup title in 2008 before joining the senior national team the same year. He has scored more than 80 international centuries and became the fastest player to reach multiple run milestones in one-day internationals. In the 2023 ICC Cricket World Cup, he scored 765 runs, the most in a single tournament, and was named Player of the Tournament. As captain of India (2014–2022), he led the team to its first Test series victory in Australia (2018–19) and maintained top ra

William Porter is an author who entered the public spotlight for writing books explaining alcohol and nicotine through physiological and psychological mechanisms. He published *Alcohol Explained* (2015) and *Alcohol Explained 2* (2019), which examine how alcohol affects the brain, sleep, anxiety, and physical dependence. He later wrote *Nicotine Explained* (2020) and co-authored *This Naked Mind: Nicotine* (2023), extending his work to tobacco and vaping. Before his writing career, he worked as a solicitor and served as a paratrooper. His books have been widely distributed and referenced in educational and wellness contexts.

William Regal is a professional wrestler and talent scout who debuted in 1983 and gained prominence in World Championship Wrestling as Lord Steven Regal, winning the WCW World Television Championship four times. He later joined WWE, where he held the Intercontinental, European, Hardcore, and World Tag Team Championships and won the 2008 King of the Ring tournament. After retiring from in-ring competition, he moved into developmental and executive roles, serving as the on-screen general manager of NXT (2014–2022) and working as a mentor and talent scout. He later returned to WWE in 2023 in a senior talent development role.

Zac Brown is a singer, songwriter, and bandleader who formed the Zac Brown Band in 2002 and broke through with the album *The Foundation* (2008), certified 5× Platinum by the RIAA. The album produced four consecutive No. 1 singles on Billboard's Hot Country Songs chart: "Chicken Fried," "Toes," "Highway 20 Ride," and "Free." He followed with No. 1 country albums including *You Get What You Give* (2010) and *Uncaged* (2012), the latter winning the Grammy Award for Best Country Album. Zac Brown Band has won three Grammy Awards and maintained a major touring presence with multiple chart-topping releases into the 2020s.

Zac Efron is an actor and producer who became widely known as Troy Bolton in Disney's *High School Musical* films (2006–2008), including the theatrical release *High School Musical 3: Senior Year* (2008), which grossed about $252.9 million worldwide. He later starred in films including *17 Again* (2009), *Neighbors* (2014), *Baywatch* (2017), *The Greatest Showman* (2017), *The Iron Claw* (2023), and *Ricky Stanicky* (2024). In 2020 he created and hosted the Netflix travel series *Down to Earth with Zac Efron*, winning the 2021 Daytime Emmy Award for Outstanding Daytime Program Host.

Zendaya is an actor, singer, and producer who first gained visibility on Disney Channel's Shake It Up (2010–2013), later starring in the TV movie *Zapped* (2014) and competing on *Dancing with the Stars* (2013). In 2017 she joined the Marvel Cinematic Universe as MJ in *Spider-Man: Homecoming* and returned in *Far From Home* (2019) and *No Way Home* (2021). She co-starred in *The Greatest Showman* (2017) and *Dune* (2021) and *Dune: Part Two* (2024). Beginning in 2019 she starred in HBO's *Euphoria* and served as an executive producer, winning Primetime Emmys (2020, 2022) and a Golden Globe (2023) for the role, becoming the youngest two-time winner for Lead Actress in a Drama Series. She produced and starred in *Challengers* (2024).

Author's Related Work

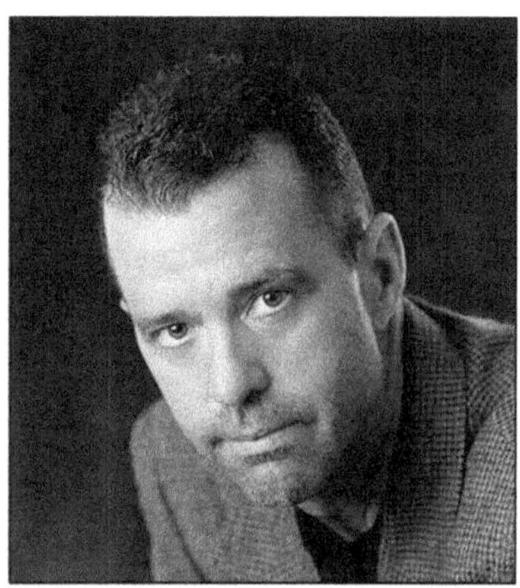

The Wealthy Gardener
Lessons on Prosperity Between Father and Son.

A timeless classic of life lessons written by a financially free father for his ambitious 20-year-old son, this book unexpectedly broke into the Top 50 of Amazon sales due to word-of-mouth referrals alone. Penned as a story about much more than wealth, you'll discover a key chapter on the **"straight edge advantage,"** which testifies to the author's own decision to quit drinking due to midlife responsibilities. You'll learn how this decision affected his future prosperity within five years. This book is a guide to mastering key principles that lead to a wealthy life.

Five-Year Crusade
The Easy Way to Achieve Your Impossible Goals.

The sequel to *The Wealthy Gardener, The 5-Year Crusade* is a book of daily actions and habits behind audacious lifetime achievement. It explains, in fictional format, the essential daily lifestyle of success combined with a habit tracker app for accountability. When you stop drinking, you will want routines in your new life. An integral part of the 5-Year Crusade system a daily checklist which includes a **30-day habit fast** to "unlearn" vices that feel good in the moment but harm you in the long run. This book outlines the small daily actions and habits that cultivate your inner power and free your potential from shackles.

Daily Crusade: A Year of Meditations for High Achievers.

Every page in this book offers a thought and an inspiring meditation designed to nurture your soul and the cultivate the *Power Within* as you strive for your best life. A repeated theme of the meditations is becoming more yourself by unlearning vices like **alcohol use or dependence.** Though originally written as a supportive work for readers of *The 5-Year Crusade*, it's gained popularity as a stand-alone book for any person willing to work for important life changes.

The Crusader's Planner: A Weekly System for High Achievers

A weekly planner that coordinates daily affirmations with the readings and meditations found in *Daily Crusade*, this book is used for journaling and tracking the small actions of the 5-Year Crusade system. Most use it is a tool to prioritize the most important "impact activities and hours" of the upcoming week. If we don't have the most important things to do every day, based on our long-term priorities, we're just dreaming. This book will help us stay accountable to our work.

Wealth Quotes: Seeds from the Garden

This is a quote book extracted from luminaries throughout history on wealth, prosperity, time, potential, and many topics related to the creation of one's best effort in life. It also contains quotes pulled from the book *The Wealthy Gardener* to serve as a refresher of the key concepts, principles, and daily mindset of a prosperous lifestyle.

The Last Word

My intention for this book was to shine a light on some extraordinary people who navigated difficult struggles and came out on top. In reading through the profiles of the stars who quit drinking, I cannot think of any word except "wow!" What an interesting group of human beings. If ever you questioned your own relationship with alcohol, know that you are in great company. I imagined this book to be a volume of quotes that would be read repeatedly to develop new references and empowering beliefs to quit drinking. I also envisioned this book to be a work that is always under construction. If a famous person catches your attention with their courageous decision to tell why they quit drinking, please share their name with me. I read every email sent to john@wealthygardener.com. I would love to include new inspiring stories in the next revision. In a sense, this book was written by the stars who told their stories with nothing to gain from the vulnerability; most of them spoke to help others with their stories. To follow their example, I will donate all royalties to promote this anthology; that is, I promise to recycle 100 percent of the book profits to expose it to the next generation of extraordinary nondrinkers. If this book helped you as a reader, please help others with your word-of-mouth referral. Or maybe just give them your book as a gift. At least give it an honest review. Thank you in advance.

John Soforic

Now What?

Research suggests that we forget 90 percent of what we read within a few weeks. If you want to make these quotes a part of your psychology, review these pages until they become embedded. These quotes are references on alcohol, and references can become empowering beliefs, which of course can become drivers of future behavior. Many former drinkers tell us that a key to their ongoing sobriety is listening to the stories of other former drinkers. Also, if you want a new direction (you are likely reading this quote book due to the pull of your soul), check out hundreds of quotes at wealthygardener.com. At this website, you will find favorite quotes listed for you to review (lesson by lesson). If you are considering a mindset shift to make a meaningful change in your life, consider the audiobook version of *The Wealthy Gardener*, narrated by Dennis Kleinman. It reached No. 46 on Amazon due to word-of-mouth referrals. This 432-page book has been described as containing the wisdom of every prosperity book in one volume. Try the free sample of the audiobook before you buy it. Check out the online reviews to see what others say. Without alcohol in your life, you will need an outlet for your emerging energy, clarity, and motivation. *The Wealthy Gardener* gives you the mindset and direction, in story format, to replace old behaviors with more purposeful actions, one day at a time.

The Wealthy Bookheads

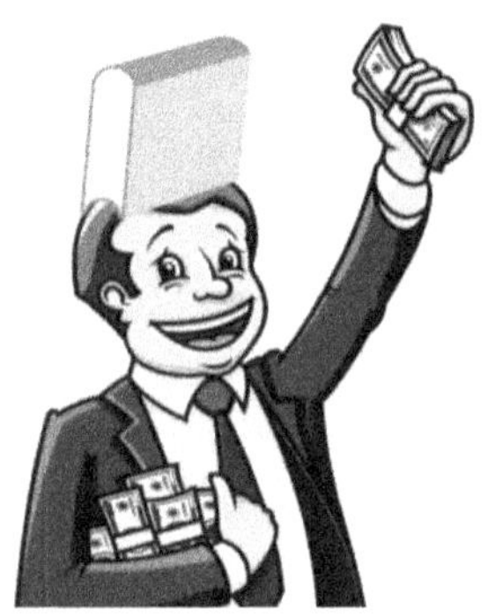

When you stop drinking, you will start growing emotionally, mentally, and spiritually. Check out wealthybookheads.com to be a lifelong learner and student of wisdom. Here you'll find a small but growing library of "book interviews." We ask the questions and let the books do the talking. We also send mini lessons to wealthy bookhead members. It's free to be a wealthy bookhead where books talk back!

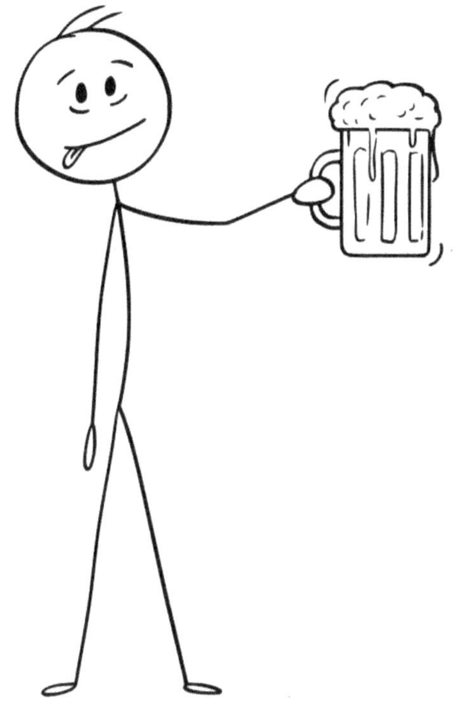

Breaking up With Booze

These stars who quit drinking come from varied professions, backgrounds, and social environments. Some of them quit drinking just to feel better in the mornings. Some of them stopped drinking to eliminate a destructive addiction. Some of them never engaged in drinking at all. What these big personalities all tell us—every single one of them quoted in these pages—is that life is better without booze.

www.ingramcontent.com/pod-product-compliance
Lightning Source LLC
Chambersburg PA
CBHW051949150726
47999CB00004B/1313